Contact Lens Fitting Guide

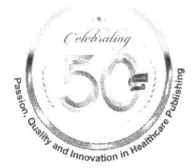

Contact Lens Fitting Guide

Second Edition

Ajay Kumar Bhootra

B Optom DOS FAO FOAI FCLI
ICLEP FIACLE (Australia)
Diploma in Sportvision (UK)
Ex - CEO and Dean
Krishnalaya School of Optometry
Kolkata, West Bengal, India

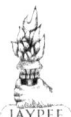

JAYPEE BROTHERS MEDICAL PUBLISHERS
The Health Sciences Publisher
New Delhi | London

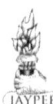 **Jaypee Brothers Medical Publishers (P) Ltd**

Headquarters
Jaypee Brothers Medical Publishers (P) Ltd
4838/24, Ansari Road, Daryaganj
New Delhi 110 002, India
Phone: +91-11-43574357
Fax: +91-11-43574314
Email: jaypee@jaypeebrothers.com

Overseas Office
J.P. Medical Ltd
83 Victoria Street, London
SW1H 0HW (UK)
Phone: +44 20 3170 8910
Fax: +44 (0)20 3008 6180
Email: info@jpmedpub.com

Website: www.jaypeebrothers.com
Website: www.jaypeedigital.com

© 2020, Jaypee Brothers Medical Publishers

The views and opinions expressed in this book are solely those of the original contributor(s)/author(s) and do not necessarily represent those of editor(s) of the book.

All rights reserved. No part of this publication may be reproduced, stored or transmitted in any form or by any means, electronic, mechanical, photocopying, recording or otherwise, without the prior permission in writing of the publishers.

All brand names and product names used in this book are trade names, service marks, trademarks or registered trademarks of their respective owners. The publisher is not associated with any product or vendor mentioned in this book.

Medical knowledge and practice change constantly. This book is designed to provide accurate, authoritative information about the subject matter in question. However, readers are advised to check the most current information available on procedures included and check information from the manufacturer of each product to be administered, to verify the recommended dose, formula, method and duration of administration, adverse effects and contraindications. It is the responsibility of the practitioner to take all appropriate safety precautions. Neither the publisher nor the author(s)/editor(s) assume any liability for any injury and/or damage to persons or property arising from or related to use of material in this book.

This book is sold on the understanding that the publisher is not engaged in providing professional medical services. If such advice or services are required, the services of a competent medical professional should be sought.

Every effort has been made where necessary to contact holders of copyright to obtain permission to reproduce copyright material. If any have been inadvertently overlooked, the publisher will be pleased to make the necessary arrangements at the first opportunity. The **CD/DVD-ROM** (if any) provided in the sealed envelope with this book is complimentary and free of cost. **Not meant for sale.**

Inquiries for bulk sales may be solicited at: jaypee@jaypeebrothers.com

Contact Lens Fitting Guide
First Edition: **2014**
Second Edition: **2020**

ISBN: 978-93-89587-10-4

Dedicated to

The entire community of Optometrists and my two loving sons, who have been my best companions. They have given me the drive and discipline to tackle any task with enthusiasm and determination.

Preface to the Second Edition

This edition of the book was driven by the desire to make it more student-friendly and comprehensive resource material. The first objective was to add questions for brainstorming. Next was to incorporate more practice associated topics, whilst at the same time maintaining the preciseness and conciseness of the book. In pursuance of this, I have added two new chapters to this edition – Contact Lens Care & Maintenance, and Sports and Contact Lenses. In addition, few more topics have been added within the existing chapters, to make the book more informative.

There is no dearth of books and resources on Contact Lenses in the market. Nonetheless, the book is unique in two ways—first, the addition of multiple-choice questions is an ambitious approach to honing the problem-solving skills of the readers, and needless to say, a great and universally used medium to test what one reads in the book. And second, a dedicated chapter on fitting contact lenses to athletes and players has been added, which is something not much seen in Contact Lens books. Sports Vision Optometry has always been one of my most favorite subjects. It is a specialized branch of Optometry. A sports vision optometrist does not work with patients for immediate remedial treatment; instead, he understands the visual deficiency of athletes and players, and tries to establish a link with his sporting performance and works with them together with coach and trainer, to improve the relevant visual skill so as to improve the their sporting performance. I dedicate this chapter to my preceptor, Prof. Geraint Griffiths.

Along with these additions, the book still maintains its original essence—it is simple, precise, and an instant reference material on the shelf. I hope it serves the purpose for which it has been written. Any suggestions for further additions and improvements to the book are always welcome.

Ajay Kumar Bhootra

Preface to the First Edition

Over the last 30 years, a lot of technological advancements have occurred in the field of optometry and ophthalmology. The corporate world has also changed. Business today has become highly networked. Patients and clients do not want to spend time in waiting. Practitioners also spend most of their time to work to retain their patients. In the process, they do not find any time to go back to the thick books to recapitulate the basic guidelines. This implies short, to-the-point guide books are very important today than ever before. Although they cannot replace the textbooks, they are a great help at the critical moment.

The idea of *Contact Lens Fitting Guide* has been conceived to serve this purpose and to create a source which is readily available with the eye care practitioners in their bag. The book is designed to have the relevant texts so that the reader can assess the key information quickly. Each chapter deals with the sequential steps needed for a particular type of contact lens. Meticulous planning has been done to design the contents and put them in an organized manner. However, the readers must take the help of other textbooks available on the subject to get into the depth.

I hope it will serve the purpose for which it has been written. I would like to welcome your suggestions to improve it further.

Ajay Kumar Bhootra

Acknowledgments

As far as I understand no creation in this world is a solo effort. Neither is this book. I have received enormous inputs of several persons from the time I conceived the idea of this book to its present shape. I would like to acknowledge everybody's effort and would like to thank all of them for bringing it to this shape. Special thanks to:

- My readers and students for their support and love
- God, who cares for me
- My amazing list of patients and clients because of whom I could have so varied experience.
- All my trainers and coaches who had been instrumental in providing me training on different occasions
- My friends and family members
- And all the people I met during my working experience and trainings who helped me understand my subject
- Above all, all the members of my organization Himalaya Optical

I am fond of reading books on various subjects. That is why while reading this book you may notice that the contents of this book are influenced by several books. Probably, that makes the disc rolls in favor of the book.

And finally, I would like to re-collect my old memories when I had my mentor Late Sri K K Binani who taught me, encouraged me, and believed in me.

Contents

1. **Introduction to Contact Lenses** **1**

   Classifications   1
   - Daily Disposable Lenses   1
   - Bi-weekly Disposable Lenses   2
   - Monthly Disposable Lenses   2
   - Traditional Lenses   3
   - Soft Hydrogel Lenses   3
   - Silicone Hydrogel Lenses   3
   - Rigid Gas Permeable Lenses   3
   - Color Cosmetic Contact Lenses   4
   - Daily Wear   4
   - Flexi Wear   4
   - Extended Wear   4
   - Continuous Wear   4

   Contact Lens Design Variables   4
   - Front and Back Surface   5
   - Overall Diameter   5
   - Base Curve   6
   - Peripheral Curves   6
   - Center Thickness   7
   - Optical Zone   7
   - Edge Design   7
   - Blending   8
   - Sagittal Height   8
   - Lenticular Zone   9
   - Contact Lens Power   9
   - Tear Lens   9

   General Properties of Contact Lens Material   10
   - Oxygen Permeability   10
   - Wettability   11
   - Biocompatibility   12
   - Water Content   12
   - Modulus of Elasticity   13
   - Ionic Charge   13

   Multiple Choice Questions   14

2. Precontact Lens Fitting Eye Examination 16

History Taking 17
Eyelids 18
   Normal 18
   Function 18
   Eyelids Examination 18
   Observe 18
   Rule Out 18
Eyelashes 19
   Normal 19
   Function 19
   Eyelash Examination 19
   Observe 19
   Rule Out 19
Lid Margin 19
   Normal 19
   Function 19
   Examination of Lid Margin 19
   Observe 19
   Rule Out 20
Cornea 20
   Normal 20
   Function 20
   Examination of Cornea 20
   Observe 20
   Rule Out 20
Conjunctiva 21
   Normal 21
   Function 21
   Examination of Conjunctiva 21
   Observe 22
   Rule Out 22
Lid Eversion 22
   Normal 22
   Lid Eversion Examination 22
   Observe 22
   Rule Out 22
Tear Film 23
   Normal 23
   Function 23
   Examination of Tear Film 23

Other Ocular Measurements 25
   Corneal Curvature 25
   Corneal Diameter 26
   Pupil Diameter 27
   Palpebral Aperture 27
   Blink Rate 28
   Lid Tonicity 28
   Corneal Sensitivity 28
   Iris Color 29
   Refraction 29

Contraindications for Contact Lens Fitting 29
Multiple Choice Questions 30

3. Fitting Soft Contact Lenses 32

Indications 32
Fitting Methods 32
Initial Data Gathering 33
   Total Lens Diameter 33
   Initial Base Curve 33
   Back Vertex Power of the Trial Lens 33

Trial Lens Selection 34
Fitting Assessment 34
   Corneal Coverage 34
   Lens Centration 35
   Lens Movement 35
   Lens Tightness 35
   Comfort 36
   Vision Stability 37
   Lens Delivery 37

Altering Soft Contact Lens Parameters 37
   Changing Total Lens Diameter 37
   Changing Back Optic Zone Radius 38

Soft Contact Lens Care System 38
   Cleaning 38
   Rinsing 38
   Disinfecting 39
   Lubricating 39
   Deproteinizing 39
   Contact Lens Case Cleaning 39

Fitting Silicone Hydrogel Lenses 41
    Base Curve Selection 42
    Movement Test 42
    Trial Method 42
    Dispense the Lens 42
    Silicone Hydrogel Lens Care System 43
Fitting Disposable Soft Contact Lenses 44
Soft Contact Lens Fitting in Dry Eyes 44
Instructions for Soft Lens Insertion 44
Instructions for Soft Lens Removal 45
Multiple Choice Questions 45

4. Fitting Soft Toric Lenses 48

Indications 48
Classification of Astigmatism (Table 4.1) 49
Fitting Methods 50
Rotational Behavior 51
Measuring Lens Rotation 52
Compensating for the Lens Rotation 53
Selecting a Toric Stabilization Design 54
    Prism Ballast 54
    Double Slab off Stabilization Design 55
    Accelerated Stability Design 55
    The 8/4 Precision Balance Design 55
Overrefraction 57
Multiple Choice Questions 57

5. Spherical RGP Lens Fitting 59

Indications 59
Fitting Methods 59
Initial Data Gathering 60
    Lens Total Diameter Selection 60
    Initial Base Curve Selection 60
    Lens Power Selection 61
Trial Lens Selection 62
Fitting Assessment 62
    Dynamic Fit 62
    Static Fit 63

Overrefraction   65
Lens Ordering   66
Rigid Gas Permeable Lens Parameters Change
and Lens Fitting   66
   Lens Total Diameter   67
   Dynamic Fitting   67
   Static Fitting   67
   Lens Thickness   67
   Base Curve   68
   Back Optic Zone Diameter   69
RGP Lens Care and Maintenance   69
Instructions for RGP Lens Insertion   70
Instructions for Rigid Gas Permeable Lens Removal   70
Multiple Choice Questions   71

6. **Therapeutic Contact Lens Fitting 73**
Indications   73
Ocular Disorders that can be Treated with
Bandage Contact Lenses   74
   Bullous Keratopathy   74
   Exposure Keratitis   74
   Corneal Ulcer   74
   Corneal Erosion   74
   Corneal Perforations   75
   Corneal Injuries   75
   Trichiasis   75
   Postoperative   75
Other Therapeutic Indications   75
   Orthoptics   75
   Corneal Irregularities   75
   Unsightly Eyes   75
   Photophobia   76
   Orthokeratology   76
Fitting Criteria   76
Therapeutic Contact Lens Care and Maintenance   76
Multiple Choice Questions   77

7. **Presbyopia and Contact Lens Fitting 78**
Monovision Correction   78
Enhanced Monovision   78

Alternating or Translating Vision Lens Design   79
Nontranslating or Simultaneous Vision Lens Design   79
   Concentric Bifocal Lenses   80
   Diffractive Lenses   80
   Aspheric Multifocal Lenses   80
Indications for Presbyopic Contact Lens Fitting   81
Fitting Methods for Soft Contact Lenses for Presbyopic Correction   81
Initial Lens Fitting Evaluation   82
Multiple Choice Questions   83

8. Sports and Contact Lenses 84
Peripheral Awareness   84
No Prismatic Effect   85
Reduced Magnifications and Minifications   85
Safety and Cosmesis   86
   Type of Contact Lenses   86
   Modality   87
   Stability   87
   Comfort   87
   Visual Performance   87
   Fitting Criteria   88
Multiple Choice Questions   89

9. Contact Lens Care and Maintenance 90
Introduction   90
Multiple Choice Questions   93

Appendices *95*
Bibliography *97*
Index *99*

CHAPTER 1

Introduction to Contact Lenses

INTRODUCTION

Contact lenses are small disk of plastic that offers an attractive, effective and non-invasive option for sight correction without the loud look of glasses. There are many choices available as far as lens material and design are concerned for vision correction. In many cases, contact lenses are used as a substitute for glasses. Contact lens may also be used to treat certain eye diseases or to change the apparent color of the eyes. The ideal lens would fully correct the refractive error with good optics and would not produce physiological or pathological changes in the eye. This would be possible only when they are fitted by a contact lens specialist in a clinical set up and after a complete evaluation of eyes using prescribed set of equipment. The successful use of contact lens requires a strong partnership between the professional skills of the practitioner and the wearer's discipline approach.

CLASSIFICATIONS

Based on wearing modalities, contact lenses can be classified as under:

Daily Disposable Lenses

Daily disposable contact lenses are used once and when they are removed from the eyes in the night before sleep, they are thrown away in the trash. When it comes to putting something into eyes, everybody would like to be conscious about his ocular health and in that respect shorter is always better. The convenience of these lenses makes them popular with lots of people.

As soon as the contact lenses are placed on the eyes, the tear deposits start building up on the lens surface. Even the best lens care system cannot remove the entire deposits from the lens surface. Over a period of time, layers of deposits build up and protein denatures. The overall effect is noticed as reduction in wettability of the lens surface which ultimately may reduce visual acuity, increase irritation and discomfort and increases the risk of infection and allergies. Daily disposable lenses allow the wearer an opportunity to replace the lens much before the likelihood of the problem arises.

In addition, the wearer of daily disposable lenses also enjoys the following benefits:
- Excellent vision throughout the day
- No ocular health compromise
- More comfort at the end of the day
- No maintenance
- Spare lenses are always available
- Eliminates the risk of potential ocular problem
- Lower incidence of visit to practitioner.

Bi-weekly Disposable Lenses

Some people may find it difficult to afford the cost of daily disposable lenses. They may find it more economical to use two weeks contact lens modality instead. As the name suggests, these contact lenses are worn for two weeks before being discarded. Remember, they need to be removed each night, therefore, cleaning, rinsing and storing in solution filled case is mandatory. The wearer has to keep the track of dates on which a new pair was put on the eyes and the date on which day he has to throw away the same. The wearer of bi-weekly disposable lenses enjoys following benefits:
- Simpler lens care
- Back up lens available
- Less dryness
- Increased comfort
- Better vision
- Better overall satisfaction.

Monthly Disposable Lenses

Monthly disposable modality is the most popular modality and is the first lens of choice by millions of people around the world. These contact lenses can be worn for one month or as directed by the practitioner. This means that at the end of every day, you remove your lenses, store them in solution, and clean before reinserting them.

Traditional Lenses

Contact lenses may be worn for a year or longer on daily wear basis. A traditional or conventional contact lens wearer must clean them on a daily basis and store them in proper protective lens case. Daily cleaning, rinsing, disinfection, and protein tablet deproteinizing are all very critical to ensure trouble-free wearing.

Contact lenses can also be classified on the basis of material type:

Soft Hydrogel Lenses

Soft contact lenses are made with a stable, solid polymer component that can absorb or bind water. Poly hydroxyethyl methacrylate (HEMA) is used to manufacture soft hydrogel lens. The lenses are made in their dry state and then hydrated in saline solution where they absorb water. The water so absorbed gives the lens its softness and makes them comfortable and pliable. Water content also increases its oxygen permeability. On an average, water content varies from 38-80%. Higher water content makes a lens less durable.

Silicone Hydrogel Lenses

Silicone hydrogel lens material is a combination of silicone rubber and hydrogel polymer. The silicone phase facilitates oxygen transmission and the hydrogel phase allows good lens movement and fluid transport. Silicone hydrogel lens materials are very different from other class of contact lens material and within the silicone hydrogel class itself major difference exists as well. The hydrogel lens materials are more of a single material family. They behave more homogenously and in that increased water content results in improved oxygen permeability. On the other hand, silicone hydrogel materials that have been introduced so far contain a variety of polymer chemistries, surface treatments, and material properties that result in less predictable eye-lens relationships.

Rigid Gas Permeable Lenses

Rigid gas permeable (RGP) contact lenses are made of rigid plastic material and contain no water. RGP lenses permit oxygen to pass directly through the lens to the eye. Because they transmit oxygen through the material, these lenses are referred to as gas permeable. They are more durable and resistant to deposits, and generally provide a crisper vision. They tend to be less expensive over the life of the lens as they last longer than soft contact lenses. They are easier to handle and less likely to tear. However, they are not as comfortable initially as soft contacts and it may take a few weeks to get used to wearing RGP lenses.

Color Cosmetic Contact Lenses

Colored contact lenses are used to change the eye color. One can change the color of his/her eyes to match facial make up. Sometimes they are also used for therapeutic reasons. They are available in wide range of colors, crazy patterns, and appeal. They are basically worn to cater the mood and aesthetic values. Colored contact lenses are also used for masking the corneal opacities. Patients with albinism or aniridia are fitted with pinhole contact lenses and amblyopic patients with dark pupil lenses.

Contact lenses can also be classified as under:

Daily Wear

Daily wear lenses are used on daily basis during the daytime. They are removed before sleeping in the night.

Flexi Wear

Flexi wear lenses are used on daily wear basis with occasional overnight wearing.

Extended Wear

Extended wear lenses are worn up to 7 days and 6 nights at a stretch without being removed from the eyes.

Continuous Wear

Continuous wear lenses are worn up to 30 days and 29 nights at a stretch before removal.

CONTACT LENS DESIGN VARIABLES

The lens design refers to the shape, size, thickness, and curve profile of the lens (Fig. 1.1). Design variables are very important aspects while manufacturing contact lenses to make a lens that will drape the cornea very gently, giving maximum comfort right from the start and at the same time ensuring peak visual performance. Each lens design variable is a part of contact lens anatomy and plays a critical

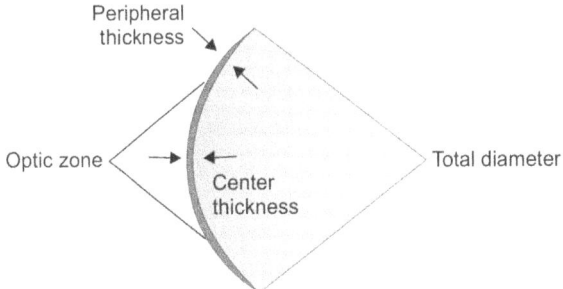

Fig. 1.1: Contact lens design variables.

part in how it functions on the eye. All of them are important and are affected by each other. These variables are:
- Front and back surface
- Overall diameter
- Base curve
- Peripheral curves
- Center thickness
- Optical zone (OZ)
- Edge design
- Blending
- Sagittal height
- Lenticular zone.

Front and Back Surface

A contact lens has two surfaces, i.e. a back surface which is in contact with the cornea and a front surface which is the surface over which the eyelids pass. The back surface of the lens is shaped to have desired relationship to the overall shape of the patient's cornea. The front surface is curved to alter the refraction of light as required for the patient's refractive error. The front surface construction may affect the action of the eyelids.

Overall Diameter

The linear measurement of the greatest distance across a lens from one outside to another outside edge, specified in millimeter is the total lens diameter. This is an important variable to determine the centration of the lens on the cornea. The corneal lenses are interlimbal or smaller in diameter, whereas corneal-scleral lenses are intermediate in size and goes beyond the corneal diameter into the sclera. Several factors determine the size of the corneal and corneal-scleral lens to be fitted. The most important is the hardness of the material. The less rigid final lens has to be bigger in size for stability of fit. The minimum functional lens diameter should be used while fitting a lens that allows adequate movement and proper position of the lens.

Base Curve

The central posterior surface curve of the contact lens is called the base curve of the contact lens and is abbreviated as BC. The other terms for the base curve include back optic zone radius (BOZR), back central optical radius (BCOR), base curve radius (BCR), and the central posterior curve (CPC). This curve is always concave and is expressed in millimeters of radius. A longer radius of curvature produces a flatter base curve and a shorter radius produces a steeper curve. The BC is the curvature from which all the curves of a lens are determined in arriving at the final dioptric power. Radiuscope is the most commonly used instrument to measure base curve of the contact lenses.

The base curve may be spherical or aspherical. A spherical base curve is specified by one radius and has same curvature at all points along the curve. An aspheric curve exhibits a gradual lengthening or shortening of the radius from the center towards the edge of the lens. The aspheric curve is specified by e-value or numerical eccentricity. The larger e-value implies greater rate of flattening or lengthening from center to edge.

Peripheral Curves

The curves surrounding the base curve on the posterior lens surface are called peripheral curves. The first curve outside the base curve is called the secondary curve; and if there is another peripheral curve, it is termed as the tertiary curve. The secondary curve is also known as intermediate posterior curve. Contact lenses are designed with one or more peripheral curves that are deliberately intended to lift away from the cornea. Each peripheral curve is typically flatter than the preceding curve in order to fit better and provide proper clearance from the gradually flattening shape of the anterior cornea. Another important thing to understand is the peripheral curve width. Peripheral curve width is the overall diameter of the lens minus the OZ. The size of peripheral curve width depends upon the size of OZ.

Center Thickness

The center thickness of a lens is the distance between the anterior and posterior surface of the lens measured at the geometric center of the lens. It determines the optical power and the fit of the lens on the cornea. It is measured in millimeter using a thickness gauge. Manufacturer usually quotes the center thickness of a lens for −3.00D. The center thickness and overall thickness profile of the lens affect the fitting characteristics, oxygen transmissibility, comfort, and handling of the lens.

In general, larger diameter requires greater thickness to have adequate dimensional stability of the lens. If the center thickness is reduced, structural stability of the lens is decreased. Increasing the thickness of the lens will cause the lid to have a great effect on the lens and will, therefore, tend to fit more loosely. On the other hand, decreasing the thickness of the lens will cause the lens to be less affected by the upper lid and consequently, it will fit more tightly. Decrease in center thickness results in reduction of weight of the lens and pressure on the cornea, but it leads the gravitational force to move behind the lens which increases the lens adherence to cornea, resulting in less lens movement.

Optical Zone

Optical zone is the central zone of the lens, the function of which is to provide the lens with an accurate and stable refractive power. On the front surface of a single curve lens, the OZ is the entire front surface of the lens. In a lenticular cut lens, OZ is the front surface minus the carrier width. On the back surface of the lens, OZ is the total diameter of the lens minus the width of the intermediate and the posterior peripheral curve. The size of the OZ is specified in millimeter which varies with lens design and lens power. In a corneal-scleral lens, the size of the OZ varies between 6–12 mm. The size of the OZ should completely cover the pupillary size at all times. If front OZ diameter is too small, the edge of the OZ will move into the pupillary area and will result in flare.

Edge Design

The edge denotes the extreme periphery of the lens where the front and the back surface meet. It is verified by using profile analyzer or stereomicroscope. The shape of the edge is one of the most important

parameters in terms of patient comfort and acceptance of contact lenses. There are two important factors to be considered as far as edge design is considered:
1. Edge profile
2. Edge thickness.

Thicker edge may make it difficult for the upper eyelids to fold over the lens edge. Round edge profile, both anterior and posterior, provides more comfort than other edge profile.

Blending

When the junction between two curves is altered either by the addition of a very narrow curve or a series of some intermediate radius, the lens is said to be blended. Specifications of the blend present are difficult because the beginning and the end of the blended area is not easily delineated and the radius of the blending curve cannot be determined. Customarily, the blend is specified as either medium or heavy. With light blending, it is possible to see the area of the blend but with heavy blending it is usually impossible to determine the width of the blend.

Sagittal Height

Sagittal height of a lens is the perpendicular distance measured in millimeter between the apex of the BOZR and the plane of the lens edge. It is an important parameter to alter the fit of the lens and is determined by the base curve of the lens and total diameter of the lens. If the base curve is constant, increasing the diameter of the lens increases the sagittal depth and therefore, the lens fit is steeper. If the diameter is constant, increasing the base curve in millimeters decreases the sagittal height and therefore, the lens fit is flatter (Fig. 1.2).

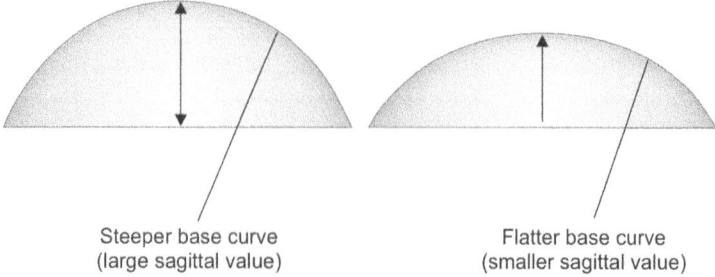

Steeper base curve (large sagittal value)   Flatter base curve (smaller sagittal value)

Fig. 1.2: Sagittal depth.

Lenticular Zone

The front surface may be divided into two zones in case of a lenticular lens design. The central zone contains the optical portion that corrects the patient's refractive error and the front peripheral zone is called the carrier. The main reason for using lenticular lens design is to reduce the thickness and weight of the lens. The carrier portion has a radius of curvature flatter than the central portion.

Contact Lens Power

Contact lenses are usually less than 0.2 mm thick and it may seem surprising that they need to be thought of as thick lenses. The thin lens formula explains the lens power as the simple addition of two surface powers. The separation of the surfaces, i.e. center thickness is assumed to be negligible and is ignored.

The contact lenses are meniscus lenses with very high surface powers. The refractive power of the lens depends on the refractive index of the material, front and back surface radii, and the lens thickness. If the lens front radius is shorter than the back surface radius, it will have plus refractive power. If the front surface radius is longer than the back surface radius, the lens has minus refractive power. The refractive power of the lens can be calculated by knowing the dimensions, but, clinically a lens power is determined directly by using the lensometer. This instrument gives the power of the contact lens in air.

Tear Lens

When a flexible lens is placed on the cornea, the "tear lens" under the contact lens is very thin. It has no dioptric power due to the conformity of the lens to the shape of the cornea. If a rigid lens is used, the tear lens depends on the relationship between the curvature of the lens back surface and the cornea (Fig. 1.3).

If the rigid lens decenters, the tear lens will acquire a prismatic component in addition to the spherical or spherocylindrical optics dictated by the fitting relationship.

Steepening the lens fit produces plus effect. So to maintain the same BVP of the system (Contact lens, tear lens, and eye), a compensating element must be added to the BVP of contact lens while ordering. Flattening the lens fit produces minus effect. So to maintain the same BVP of the system (CL, tear lens, and eye), compensating element must be added to the BVP of contact lens while ordering.

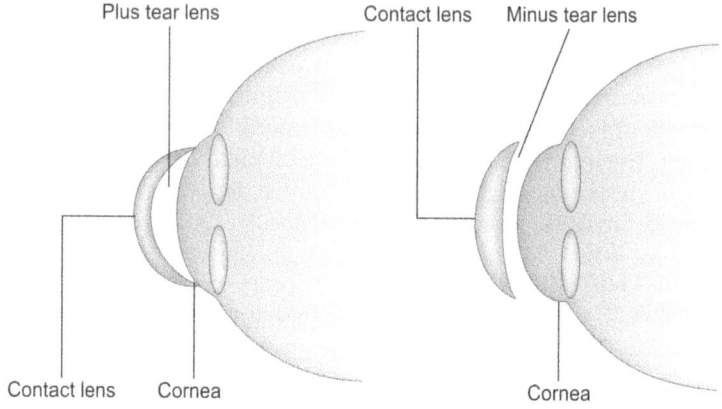

Fig. 1.3: Tear lens.

GENERAL PROPERTIES OF CONTACT LENS MATERIAL

Material properties together with surface properties influence the lens fitting on eye, wearing comfort, and oxygen permeability and may lead to ocular difficulties. The general properties of contact lens material are:

Oxygen Permeability

Corneal hypoxia has been implicated in many of the ocular complications associated with contact lens wear. In the absence of a contact lens, the oxygen required for the metabolic functioning of the cornea comes primarily from the atmosphere. The peripheral cornea may also receive some oxygen supply from the limbal vasculature, while the posterior cornea is supplied oxygen from the aqueous humor. In order to maintain normal corneal metabolism during contact lens wear and prevent hypoxia, it is necessary that any material used as a contact lens is able to allow the passage of oxygen to be maintained.

Oxygen permeability is the physical property of the material and is a measure of the oxygen performance of a lens material. However, actual amount of oxygen transmitted (Fig. 1.4) to the cornea after putting on the contact lenses depend also upon the lens thickness which is the important feature of finished contact lenses. Manufacturers often quote permeability values and transmissibility values separately. Transmissibility is usually based on the thickness of a –3.00 lens but lenses of different back vertex powers will have different thickness and hence transmissibility. Also, for accurate

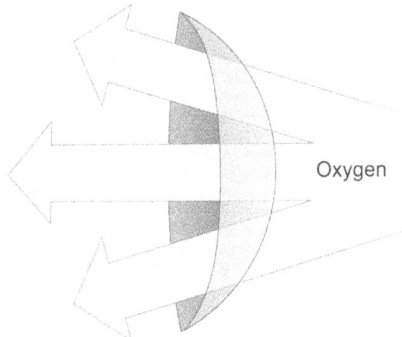

Fig. 1.4: Schematic representation of Oxygen transmission through lens.

values the measurements should be edge corrected. Water contents of the lens material and dehydration during lens wear also affect the transmissibility.

Contact lens needs to provide atmospheric oxygen to the cornea. Normal concentration of oxygen in air is 20.95%. A reduction in amount of oxygen reaching cornea through lens causes several problems, for example striae may be observed in the posterior stroma if the oxygen reaching through the lens falls below 5% or folds may be observed in the deep stroma if oxygen reaching through the lens falls below 8%.

Wettability

Wettability can be thought of as the formation of a continuous fluid film over the contact lens surface. In order to achieve good vision and consistent comfort, a stable uniform tear film must be supported over the front surface of a contact lens. A lens that does not have good wetting characteristics will result in a rapid breakup of the pre-lens tear film and a consequent reduction in vision quality. A stable pre-lens tear film provides a lubricating effect, allowing comfortable lid movement over the front surface of the lens. A wettable contact lens material is more likely to allow a continuous tear film between the back surface of the lens and the corneal epithelium, which is important consideration for biocompatibility. A contact lens surface with poor wettability has a greater tendency to attract tear-film deposits. As the tear film dries out due to evaporation between blinking, the dry spots form areas prone to deposit formation, especially protein, and this in turn further reduces surface wettability.

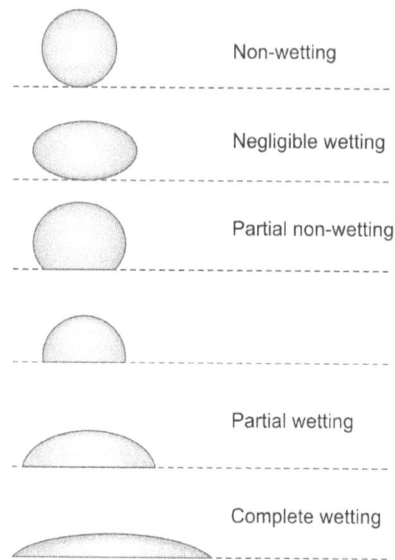

Fig. 1.5: From non-wetting to complete wetting of contact lens surface.

Traditionally, wettability can be measured by measuring the contact angles. When a drop of liquid is placed on a solid surface, an angle is formed between the surface and a tangent to the surface of the drop at the point of contact is referred to as a contact angle. The lower the angle, the more completely the liquid wets the surface (Fig. 1.5). An angle of 0° implies complete wettability, allowing the tear spread evenly over the lens surface to provide stable tear film. Clinically, it can be measured using subjective scales of tear break-up over a lens.

Biocompatibility

Since lenses come in contact with the eye, they should be considered as biomaterials, which must fulfill most of the general biological requirements of all other biomedical polymers. Specific toxicity, carcinogenicity, and sterility tests for the evaluation of biomaterials in general have been recommended.

Water Content

Water content of a lens material is the amount of the fluid taken up by the contact lens material. Most contact lens materials, both hard and soft, absorb some water. The amount absorbed is usually expressed as a percentage of total weight. Most of the material used today have water content which ranges from 38% to 79%. Contact lens with water content less than 50% is called low water content and contact lens with more than 50% water content are called high water content lenses. When a material absorbs water, it swells which makes high water content lens thicker. Higher water content materials allow more oxygen through them than the low water materials. Materials that absorb less than 4% water by weight are referred as hydrophobic and those that absorb 4% or more water are termed as hydrophilic. With hydrophilic polymers, increasing the water content generally increases the oxygen transmissibility. However, this often increases lens fragility and may make materials more prone to deposit formation.

Modulus of Elasticity

A contact lens is subject to stress because of external forces on the eye by the lids, during handling and also during the manufacturing process. The modulus of elasticity is a constant value that expresses a material's ability to keep its shape when subjected to stress. Materials with a low modulus of elasticity are less resistant to stress and they quickly conform to the shape of the eye and materials with a high modulus resist stress, hold their shape better, tend to provide better visual acuity, and easier handling. A truly elastic material is one that will return to its original shape after deformation, once the load has been removed.

Ionic Charge

Contact lens materials may possess an electrical charge or they may be electrically neutral. The electrically charged materials are called ionic and no charge materials are called nonionic. This attribute is especially important in soft hydrogel lens materials, as it affects factors such as solution compatibility and deposit formation. In most cases, contact lenses are negatively charged which causes the materials to be more reactive, especially in solutions that are acidic. This in turn can cause dimensional changes and even material degradation. It may also cause a material to be more prone to deposits formation. Nonionic materials tend to be more inert and less reactive with tear constituents, so they also tend to be more deposit resistant.

SUMMARY

Optically, contact lenses are no different as compared to other vision correction devices. However, contact lens designing is not an easy task. Fewer degrees of freedom in lens design are available. This is because the back surface of the contact lens must relate to the anterior geometry of the eye. Narrow range of refractive indices is available as it is determined by the material selected, which is usually a clinical rather than an optical decision. The lens designer often has no choice of refractive index. The range of indices within a lens type is also relatively narrow. The optical surface shape of flexible lenses is determined by conformance to corneal shape, as well as lens profile and material physical properties. The optics of RGP lenses, while more predictable, may involve noncoaxial optics due to lens movement and decentration. This means the exact effects are difficult to predict or calculate.

MULTIPLE CHOICE QUESTIONS

Q. 1. Which of the following is the advantage of daily disposable contact lenses?
 a. Reduce possibility of irritation and discomfort
 b. Reduce risk of infection and allergies
 c. Good and consistent visual acuity
 d. All of the above

Q. 2. What is the importance of overall diameter of the contact lenses while dispensing to a patient?
 a. This is an important variable to ensure the maximum comfort
 b. This is an important variable to determine the centration of contact lenses on the cornea
 c. This is important variable to determine the accurate and stable refractive power
 d. None of the above

Q. 3. What is the base curve of the contact lenses?
 a. The front surface curve is known as the base curve of the contact lenses
 b. The back surface curve is known as the base curve of the contact lenses
 c. The central posterior surface curve of the contact lenses is known as the base curve of the contact lenses
 d. The anterior posterior surface curve of the contact lenses is known as the base curve of the contact lenses

ANSWERS

| 1. d | 2. b | 3. c |

Q. 4. The central thickness and overall thickness profile of contact lenses affects:
   a. Oxygen transmissibility
   b. Wearing comfort
   c. Lens handling
   d. All of the above

Q. 5. What is likely to happen when optical zone diameter of contact lenses is smaller than the pupillary diameter of the wearer?
   a. The edge of the optical zone of the contact lens will move into the pupillary area and will result in flare
   b. The contact lens will be a tight fit
   c. The patient will have fluctuating vision
   d. All of the above

ANSWERS

4. d   5. a

CHAPTER 2

Precontact Lens Fitting Eye Examination

INTRODUCTION

A successful contact lens fitting is taken when the wearer uses the contact lens comfortably without any serious complications, follows the instructions and guidelines of his optometrist and finally replaces his old contact lens with the new one as per schedule with the same optometrist. This is possible only when comprehensive ocular examination has been conducted before fitting the lens, a suitable wearer has been fitted with the most appropriate lens for his eyes, and is being educated adequately to follow the wearing schedule, care and maintenance and replacement schedule. Precontact lens fitting examination puts the foundation stone which helps to achieve following goals:

- A baseline data for fitting contact lenses.
- Determine ocular health and suitability of contact lens wear.
- Determine best contact lens design and material, parameters of first diagnostic lens, so that the correct lens parameters can be ordered.
- Rule out unsuitable candidates.
- To be able to explain limitations and risks associated with the lens.
- Finally, establish reasonable expectations from the contact lens wear.

A comprehensive precontact lens fitting ocular examination starts with history taking and is followed by examination of following ocular structures and tests to define contact lens parameters:

- Eyelids
- Eyelashes
- Lid margin
- Cornea
- Conjunctiva
- Lid eversion
- Lid tonicity

- Corneal sensitivity
- Tear film
- Corneal curvature measurement
- Corneal diameter measurement
- Pupil diameter
- Palpebral aperture
- Blink rate
- Iris color
- Refraction.

HISTORY TAKING

History taking and understanding symptoms is probably one of the most important aspects of any medical examination and is also very critical before fitting contact lenses. It is not only important to elicit the critical points of health and visual problem, but is equally important to demonstrate your expertize and to break the barrier between you and the patient. During the process of history taking, a kind of trust is built between the patient and the practitioner. The result is that the patient starts taking your advices. The patient who intends to wear contact lenses comes to the optometrist with healthy eyes and it is, therefore, the moral duty of the optometrist to maintain the ocular health of the patient. Relevant questions should be asked which are needed to understand:

- A brief history of the general health of the potential wearer to know various conditions like allergies, diabetes, frequent cough and cold, cardiovascular problem, hormone replacement, thyroid, etc. is important to rule out unsuitable candidate for contact lens wear.
- Ocular history with respect to previous correction, ocular allergies, dry eyes, ocular injuries, previous ocular surgery, and other ocular diseases. Ocular history helps optometrist to diagnose and take treatment decision. It also helps prescribing appropriate contact lenses.
- Current list of medications is more informative than the patient's answer to questions related to his general health.
- *Known allergies*: Contacts are placed directly on the eye, where they float on the tear film in front of the cornea. A set of care regimen products are prescribed for healthy contact lens wear which contains preservatives and other ingredients. Allergy to anything may lead to chronic allergic conditions and hence drop out from the contact lens wear.

- Past contact lens history is important to determine whether the patient has worn contact lens before or not. In case the answer to this question is positive, additional questioning like since when, for how long, what type of lens, why did he discontinue, are important. The answer to these questions will help the optometrist to avoid the mistake that might have been done by the previous practitioners.
- Patient's expectations and motivational level makes sure that patient is ready to bear the cost involved and is ready to spend required time to follow the set guideline.
- Patient's hygiene is very important because success depends a lot upon patient's hygiene.

History taking is also an opportunity to explain the significance of different testing procedures that will follow to ensure his cooperation.

EYELIDS

Normal

The eyelids are modified folds of skin. They are the thinnest skin on the face.

Function

The eyelids protect the eyes from foreign bodies and sudden increase in the level of incident light. They also spread tears and aid to tear film stability.

Eyelids Examination

Use slit lamp with diffuse illumination. Set the illumination arm approximately at 30° from the straight ahead position and use low magnification.

Observe

With this set up, the optometrist should carry out several sweeps across the anterior eyelid and adnexa to look for dryness, redness, swelling, or any abnormal growth and make sure that there is absence of inflammation, normal redness and anatomy of eyelids, and smooth surface texture of lid skin.

Rule Out

Any inflammation of lids should ideally be ruled out.

EYELASHES

Normal

Eyelashes are hair that grows at the edge of the eyelid. They take 7–8 weeks to regrow if pulled out.

Function

Eyelashes protect the eyes from debris and provide attention warning when a strange object invades eyes.

Eyelash Examination

Use slit lamp with diffuse illumination. Set the illumination arm approximately at 30° from the straight ahead position and use low magnification.

Observe

With this set up, observe loss of eyelashes, their unusual position, any irregular growth, presence of crusts or scales in the lashes, and make sure the presence of hygiene.

Rule Out

Unhygienic eyelashes, irregular growth of eyelashes, or inward growth of eyelashes should be ruled out.

LID MARGIN

Normal

The lid margins are shelf-like portion of the eyelids.

Function

Lid margin acts as hot bed for metabolic activities. Secretions from glands around lid margin help maintain tear film quality.

Examination of Lid Margin

Use slit lamp with diffuse illumination. Set the illumination arm approximately at 30° from the straight ahead position and use low magnification.

Observe

With this set up, look for any redness, oiliness, and any abnormal growth. Ask the patient to open his eyes, and examine the lid margins for patency of the tear ducts and meibomian glands. Then place your index finger close to the patient's lower lid margin and evert the lower lid and scan the inferior palpebral and bulbar conjunctiva looking for elevation, depressions, or discolorations.

Rule Out

Meibomitis, blepharitis, stye, chalazia, and meibomian glands dysfunction should be ruled out.

CORNEA

Normal

Normal cornea is regular in shape, transparent, has luster, and is characterized by absence of blood vessels. Slit lamp examination shows bright corneal reflex and convex reflecting surface.

Function

The anterior cornea acts as a major refracting surface.

Examination of Cornea

Slit lamp is used to examine the cornea. The following four illumination techniques can be used:
- Diffuse broad beam for overall examination
- Parallelepiped or wide beam examination
- Narrow beam examination
- Fluorescein staining.

Observe

While examining cornea using slit lamp, look for regularity in its shape and transparency, presence of any scar, blood vessels, and corneal haze (Table 2.1).

Fluorescein staining examination is very important in contact lens practice. The appearance of fluorescein in the eye may be enhanced by placing a yellow barrier filter over eyepiece.

Rule Out

Central corneal clouding, punctate keratitis, corneal scarring, corneal striae, corneal folds, epithelial wrinkling, microcysts, etc. should be ruled out.

TABLE 2.1: Slit lamp observation.

Illumination techniques	Observe
Diffuse illumination	General view of the anterior cornea
Parallelepiped or wide beam examination	For surface and sectional study of cornea to locate the corneal lesion. A three-dimensional block of cornea can be observed which allows us to ascertain the position of any interesting feature, e.g. foreign body, corneal abrasion, etc. in the cornea.
Narrow beam examination	Narrow slit beam with high magnification allows us to see the brilliant optical section image obtained from cornea. This is used to ascertain the depth of lesion, variations in corneal curvature, and corneal thickness.
Fluorescein staining	Sodium fluorescein is a vital stain that colors the damaged epithelium tissues. It is the best means to judge corneal and conjunctival integrity. It is very useful in revealing even the minutest abrasion on the cornea.

CONJUNCTIVA

Normal

The conjunctiva is a mucous membrane consisting of loose, vascular connective tissue. It is transparent. Transparency is less than that of the cornea when observed with a slit lamp.

Function

Conjunctiva membrane lines the posterior surface of the lids and reflected onto the anterior surface of the globe.

Examination of Conjunctiva

Use slit lamp diffuse illumination with low magnification to examine the conjunctiva. Once upper and lower lid margins have been examined, the optometrist should look at the bulbar conjunctiva to assess hyperemia and the possible presence of a pinguecula or pterygium. Then examine the superior and inferior palpebral conjunctiva for hyperemia, follicles, and papillae. Then ask the patient to look down. Place your thumb close to the upper lid margin and elevate the lid. Scan across the superior bulbar conjunctiva. Instruct the patient to look first to the left and then to right, while you scan the nasal and temporal bulbar conjunctiva. Finally, evert the upper lid. It is necessary to examine the palpebral conjunctival tissue. This may reveal subtle lid changes or irritation related to contact lenses. It will also assist in the differential diagnosis of lid disease.

Observe

Observe carefully redness, swelling, or any abnormal growths.

Rule Out

Pinguecula or pterygium should be ruled out; if position of pinguecula/pterygium is close to the limbus, it may affect contact lens fit [especially rigid gas permeable (RGP)].

LID EVERSION

Normal

Upper lid eversion examination is very important in contact lens fitting. Examine palpebral conjunctival tissue, i.e. conjunctiva lining the inner eyelids and extending to the lid margins. Equally important is the lower lid retraction examination. It also assist in the differential diagnosis of lid disease.

Lid Eversion Examination

Use slit lamp diffuse illumination with low magnification to examine the conjunctiva. In order to examine palpebral conjunctiva, evert the upper lid and examine the tissue in five regional areas, i.e. upper, central, lower, nasal, and temporal regions.

The lower lid is retracted by gently pulling down the skin with the thumb or forefinger and exposing the inner palpebral conjunctiva. The patient is instructed to look up while the lower lid is held. Avoid touching the lower lid margin or applying too much pressure against the skin.

Observe

This may reveal subtle lid changes or irritation related to contact lenses. Look for any redness, swelling, roughness, abnormal growth, or concretions.

Rule Out

Giant papillary conjunctivitis, internal hordeolum, or any other abnormality should be ruled out.

TEAR FILM

Normal

The tear film is a thin layer of fluid that covers the ocular surface. It is the first refractive media striking the light rays. It is composed of three layers: lipid, aqueous, and mucin, which are secreted by glands around eyelid. Three layers serve as oil, water, and mucous. The lower mucous layer serves as an anchor for the tear film and helps it adhere to the eye. The middle layer is comprised of water. The upper oil layer seals the tear film and prevents evaporation. The tears are distributed by normal and voluntary eyelid action, with each blink "resurfacing" the precorneal tear film and also by normal and voluntary movement of the globe. Total tear volume is 6.5–8.5 microliter (ml). Aging increases the tear viscosity.

Function

Tear film keeps the eye moist, creates a smooth surface for light to pass through the eye, nourishes the front of the eye, and provides protection from injury and infection. For safe and comfortable contact lens wear, we need adequate tear volume to support eye and contact lens and good tear film quality that "clear" tears with good stability. Poor tear film may result in:
- Dry eye symptoms
- Poor lens fit
- Lens intolerance
- Reduced vision
- Tissue damage
- Infection.

Examination of Tear Film

Tear volume adequacy, stability, and regularity of tear film are important aspects of healthy tear film.
   Two kinds of tear film assessment is needed:
1. Tear volume (Schirmer Test, Tear Prism Height)
2. Tear film quality [tear break-up time (TBUT), noninvasive tear break up time (NIBUT), tear thinning time (TTT), Rose Bengal test, PRTT].

Schirmer Test

Bend the Schirmer strip at their notch and hook it over the nasal lower lid margin and ask the patient to look up before insertion of the filter strip and also during the 5-minute test. Blinking is permitted during the test.

The adequacy of tear volume is measured by the length of wet area of the filter strip measured from the notch. Values range from less than 5 mm to more than 33 mm of wetting. Normal average value is taken as 15 mm of wetting in 5 minutes. Wetting lengths less than 5 mm in 5 minutes should be viewed with suspicion.

A topical anesthetic drop may be applied to measure basal tear. Use cotton swab to remove excess tear fluid and then put the strip as used in the normal Schirmer test for 5 minutes. A normal reading is approximately 10 mm in this case.

Tear Prism Height

The height and width of tear reservoir across the lower lid margin can give a reasonable assessment of tear volume. Use slit lamp and reduce the height of slit beam and adjust to the horizontal position. The approximate height of tear prism at the center in case of normal tear film is 0.2–0.4 mm and 0.2 mm at the periphery. Reduced height suggests reduced tear volume and increased height suggests poor drainage system.

Direct observation of the tears can provide indications as to the quality of the tears, i.e. good tears generally flow briskly with blink and contain few contaminants. Debris observed in tear meniscus is at times seen in dry eyes.

Tear Break-up Time

Tear break-up time is a test to measure the relative stability of the precorneal tear film. The time required for the ocular surface to lose cohesive surface wetting after each blink is referred to as the TBUT. Due to evaporation, there is a localized thinning of the tear film which appears as dry spots formed when the film breaks up and the tears recede and is observed as black patch.

Sodium fluorescein is instilled onto the eye and the tear film is monitored under "blue light". A record is taken of the first occurrence of a "dry spot" which appears as a black area in the tear film. Care should be taken not to touch or disturb the lids, and to maintain the normal position of the lids. Break-up time (BUTs) of <10 seconds are considered abnormal and BUTs of 15–45 seconds are considered normal.

Tear Thinning Time

A keratometer is used instead of a slit lamp or a tearscope. While the blink is held, the keratometer's mire images are observed and the time of the first image disturbance is noted. Any image disturbance is attributed to alterations of the tear film. Shorter times than BUT have been reported, suggesting a greater sensitivity to tear film changes.

Lipid Layer Thickness Assessment

Lipid layer thickness (LLT) controls the rate of evaporation of the deeper aqueous layer, tear film stability, and also dry eyes symptoms. Thicker LLT is desirable. Assessment of LLT have been correlated with examining the color interference patterns. Numerous methods of utilizing interference patterns have been used to measure LLT, including slit lamp and others. Different patterns like color fringes, amorphous, flow pattern, or open meshwork may be observed as an indicator of lipid layer thickness.

OTHER OCULAR MEASUREMENTS

The examination of anterior segment of the eye is necessary to discover any condition that would exclude contact lens wear. In addition, certain ocular measurements are needed to determine the fitting parameters of the contact lenses. These include following ocular measurements:

- Corneal curvature
- Corneal diameter
- Pupil diameter
- Palpebral aperture
- Blink rate
- Lid tonicity
- Corneal sensitivity
- Iris color
- Refraction.

Corneal Curvature

Keratometer is used to measure corneal curvature which helps to select base curvature of initial diagnostic lens to try on the cornea to assess the fit. This is especially important in case of RGP lens fitting. Keratometer gives radius of curvature which may be converted into corneal diopter by using following formula:

$$D = \frac{(n-1) \times 1000}{r}$$

Where r is radius of curvature in mm and n is the refractive index of cornea, which is taken as 1.3375.

The lower and upper limits of keratometer readings are 6.40 mm and 9.40 mm.

Corneal Diameter

Corneal diameter is measured with reference to horizontal visible iris diameter (HVID) and vertical visible iris diameter (VVID). Use simple mm scale to measure HVID and VVID and add 2 mm to HVID to select the lens diameter of initial soft contact trial lens and subtract 2 mm for the RGP trial lens selection. Normal HVID and VVID are 11.7 mm and 10.6 mm, respectively (Figs. 2.1 and 2.2).

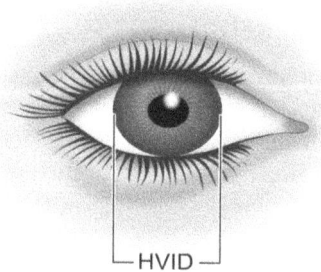

Fig. 2.1: HVID measurement.

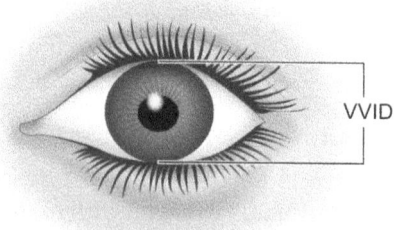

Fig. 2.2: VVID measurement.

Pupil Diameter

Pupil diameter is measured in dim light with simple mm scale and 1 mm is added to the measurement in order to decide the back optic zone diameter (BOZD) of the contact lens (Fig. 2.3).

Palpebral Aperture

Palpebral aperture is measured with a millimeter rule from the upper lid margin to the lower lid margin across the center of the pupil while the eye is in the relaxed primary gaze position. Average palpebral aperture size in noncontact lens wearer is 10.10 mm (Fig. 2.4).

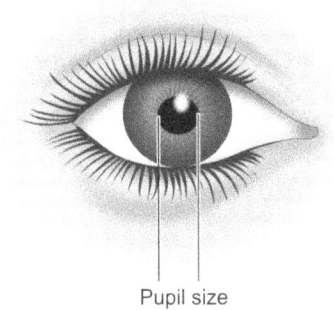

Fig. 2.3: Pupil diameter.

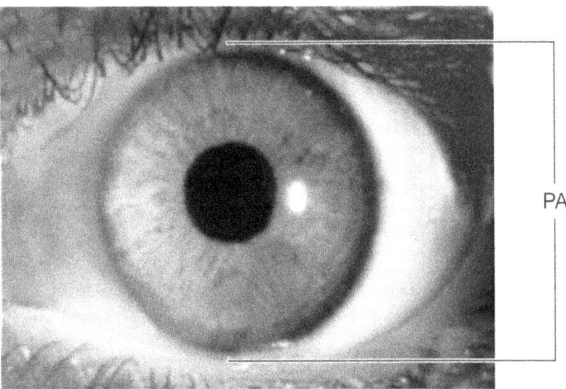

Fig. 2.4: Palpebral aperture size.

Blink Rate

An adequate blink rate is necessary to prevent desiccation of the ocular surface. Partial blinking may result in superficial punctate staining of the cornea.
- Normal blink rate is 15 blinks/minute.
- 22 blinks/minute during relaxed condition.
- 18 blinks/minute during conversation.
- 10 blinks/minute while reading a book.
- 7 blinks/minute while viewing text on computer display.
- 4 blinks/minute during extensive computer use.

Normal blink rate should be measured whilst talking to the patient without alerting him to what is being done. Awareness may invalidate the results. A blink usually lasts for 0.3 seconds.

How to measure blink rate?
- Normal lit room
- Patient not sitting under fan or in front of air condition draft
- No bright light on patient's eyes
- Practitioner sitting right in front of the patient
- Stop watch in hand
- Do not say anything to the patient
- Keep your eyes on patient's eyes
- Count the number of times patient blinks
- Also note blink type.

Lid Tonicity

Lid tension significantly influences lens centration and movement for both rigid and soft lenses. Higher lid tensions cause greater lens displacement on blinking. A large diameter RGP lens with a thick minus carrier may ride high under a tight upper lid, while a smaller diameter lens may be pushed down. No accurate method of measuring lid tension exists. Ask the patient to look down, pull the upper lid outward by grasping the eyelashes gently, and subjectively grade the resistance to pulling from very tight to very loose.

Corneal Sensitivity

Corneal sensitivity refers to the capability of the cornea to respond to stimulation. Corneal sensitivity varies across the cornea, with center being the most sensitive. Ocular diseases and rigid contact lens wear greatly reduce the sensitivity of the cornea. Aging and the presence of arcus senilis also leads to reduction in corneal sensitivity. In diabetic

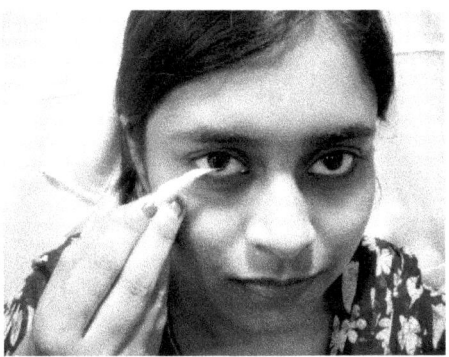

Fig. 2.5: Corneal sensitivity test.

patients, corneal sensitivity is reduced due to loss of corneal nerve fibers. Clinically, corneal sensitivity can be measured with the wisp of cotton (Fig. 2.5). All the quadrants are tested with the eyeball rotated downward, upward, nasally, and laterally.

Iris Color

The iris color should be recorded for prosthetic or cosmetic lens fitting.

Refraction

Vision correction is the main goal for fitting contact lenses for which complete objective and subjective refraction is needed and visual acuity is measured. Complete distance refraction is to be followed by near vision correction. The results of sphero-cylinder refraction is converted into spherical equivalent for spherical lens fitting and is compensated for vertex distance to derive the results at corneal plane.

CONTRAINDICATIONS FOR CONTACT LENS FITTING

- Frequent upper respiratory tract infections. This involves acute infection involving nose, sinuses, pharynx, or larynx. Viral conjunctivitis is often associated with it. Contact lens wearer should be informed of potential risk of contact lens induced acute red eye (CLARE).
- Allergies such as hay fever, asthma, allergic rhinitis. People with these conditions are prone to itchy and watery eyes.
- Dermatological problems such as atopic eczema, psoriasis, and acne rosacea.

- In insulin dependent diabetes, corneal epithelium may be more fragile and can delay healing response.
- *Immunosuppressive drugs,* drugs inhibit or prevent activity of immune system.
- Thyroid dysfunction causes dryness.
- In pregnancy, hormonal changes can disturb the tear film and water retention causes edema that changes the curvature of cornea.
- Very anxious, nervous, or impatient individual may not be accepting compromises in comfort, vision, or time required for lens care.
- Poor compliant patient.
- Person with poor hygiene.
- *Chronic alcoholic patients*: They are usually confronted with sore eyes.
- Active ocular diseases such as keratitis, conjunctivitis, iritis, etc.
- If the patient has a history of recurrent ocular disease such as iritis, ulcer, conjunctivitis, recurrent erosions, etc. then the patient should not be fitted with contact lenses.
- Corneal neovascularization or ghost vessels may be reactivated with contact lens wear.
- Blepharitis and meibomianitis increase chances of infection.

MULTIPLE CHOICE QUESTIONS

Q. 1. What has been suggested as the normal blink rate?
 a. 6 blinks/minute
 b. 12 blinks/minute
 c. 15 blinks/minute
 d. 8 blinks/minute

Q. 2. What is considered to be the average HVID?
 a. 11.70 mm
 b. 12.70 mm
 c. 11.90 mm
 d. 13.50 mm

Q. 3. Which slit lamp technique is used to view eye lashes and lid margins?
 a. Diffuse illumination
 b. Specular reflection
 c. Sclerotic scatter
 d. Retro illumination

ANSWERS

| 1. c | 2. a | 3. a |

Q. 4. How is sectional examination of cornea done to locate corneal lesion with the help of slit lamp?
a. Using parallelepiped technique
b. Using narrow slit beam
c. Using diffuse illumination
d. Using direct illumination

Q. 5. How is tear film quality assessed?
a. Using Schirmer test
b. Using tear prism height
c. Using tear break up time
d. All of the above

Q. 6. Which of the following represents the normal tear prism height?
a. 0.2 mm
b. 0.1–0.3 mm
c. 0.2–0.4 mm
d. 0.3 mm

Q. 7. How is tear volume assessed?
a. Using Schirmer test
b. Using NIBUT
c. Using tear break up time
d. Rose Bengal test

Q. 8. While fitting contact lens to a patient how is BOZD of initial contact lens determined?
a. Pupil diameter as measured in dim light
b. Pupil diameter as measured in full room light
c. Pupil diameter as measured in dim light plus 1 mm
d. Pupil diameter as measured in full room light minus 1 mm

Q. 9. What is the significance of assessing lid tonicity while fitting contact lenses to a patient?
a. Lid tonicity influences lens centration and lens movement on eye
b. Lid tonicity influences overall lens diameter
c. Lid tonicity influences subjective wearing comfort
d. None of the above

Q. 10. What is suggested as the oxygen requirement of the cornea to prevent corneal sensitivity loss?
a. 8%
b. 6%
c. 10%
d. 4%

Q. 11. Which of the following has been suggested as the contraindication for contact lenses?
a. Poor compliant patient
b. Patient with poor hygiene
c. A very anxious, nervous, and impatient person
d. All of the above

ANSWERS

4. a	5. c	6. c	7. a	8. c
9. a	10. a	11. d		

Chapter 3

Fitting Soft Contact Lenses

INTRODUCTION

The soft contact lens (SCL) assumes the shape of the cornea as they drape over the corneal surface. They are fitted larger than the horizontal measurement of visible iris diameter and flatter than the cornea. Fluorescein is likely to stain the lenses and hence it is not the usual practice to use fluorescein to check the fitting of SCLs. Some practitioners occasionally use high molecular sodium fluorescein for the purpose.

INDICATIONS

- Spherical SCL are indicated for almost all spherical corneas.
- Soft contact lenses are the first choice when the comfort is the important criteria.
- As far as astigmatic errors are concerned, some practitioners are of opinion to fit spherical SCLs when the amount of astigmatic error is less than equal to 0.75 D.
- Soft contact lenses are also the lens of choice when there is significant corneal astigmatism but manifest refraction is spherical. Fitting rigid lens may induce residual astigmatism in such cases.

FITTING METHODS

There are two philosophies of fitting SCLs. They are:
- Empirical method
- Trial lens fitting method.

Under empirical method, the optometrist obtains the lens prescription, corneal curvature, and lens diameter and does not put any trial lens on the patient's eyes; he gets the lens from the laboratory and informs the patient when it is ready. The patient does not get the feel of the lens before the final lens is delivered to him. Contrarily, under trial lens fitting method, the optometrist follows a sequential step of SCL fitting philosophy which includes initial data gathering, trial lens selection, and fitting assessment before the final lens is ordered to laboratory.

INITIAL DATA GATHERING

The optometrist needs to collect certain basic information to select initial trial lens to be put on the patient's eyes for fitting assessment with respect to lens total diameter (TD), initial base curve, and lens power. Care should be taken to ensure that the first lens placed on the patient's eye guides you to the final fit.

Total Lens Diameter

Lens diameter is one of the most important parameters for the successful SCL fitting. In order to decide the lens diameter, simply measure HVID with simple mm scale and then add 2 mm to the horizontal visible iris diameter (HVID) or follow the manufacturer's recommendations. Consider larger diameter for higher prescription, higher water content lenses, and flatter corneas. Also measure BOZD, i.e. back optic zone diameter. The normal BOZD is taken in the range of 8–11 mm which varies with back vertex power (BVP) of the lens—smaller with higher prescription.

Initial Base Curve

The selection of the back optic zone radius (BOZR) or base curve of the initial trial lens is done, based upon keratometry reading. Take the two K-readings, either add 0.8 mm to flatter K, or, add 1.00 mm to average K, or select 4.00 D flatter than average K, or follow the manufacturer's recommendations. BOZR is relatively unimportant in case of very thin lenses, but is important for thicker lenses.

Back Vertex Power of the Trial Lens

A complete subjective refraction has to be done and the results are used to find out the spherical equivalent. If a patient has low astigmatic error, spherical equivalent will most likely provide clearer vision. Then compensate the results nearest to vertex distance correction. Vertex distance compensation is very significant when the refractive error is more than 4.00 D. The following formula is used for finding the spherical equivalent:

Spherical equivalent = Sphere + ½ of the astigmatic error

The vertex distance compensation formula is as under:

$$F(cl) = \frac{F(Sp)}{1-dF(Sp)}$$

Where d stands for change in vertex distance in meters.

For example, a given spectacle refraction reads $-7.00/-1.00 \times 180$
Spherical equivalent $= (-7.00) + (-0.50) = -7.50$ D

Contact lens power after vertex correction will be:

$$F(cl) = \frac{-7.50}{1-(+0.012)(-7.50)} = -6.88 \text{ Dsph}$$

The nearest contact lens available in the trial set will be -7.00 Dsph.

TRIAL LENS SELECTION

Once the initial data has been gathered, the first trial lens should be selected in such a way so that it may guide us to the final lens fit. Select the trial lens from the trial set which is close to the vertex compensated correction. If the power difference is more, then it is always possible to have mismatch in the final lens fitting as compared to trial lens fitting. The initial base curve of the trial lens should be based on the K-reading and lens TD has to be 2 mm larger than the HVID measurement. Before inserting the trial lens into the patient's eyes, the practitioner must counsel the patient regarding the sensation he will notice when the lens will be placed on the cornea. Ask the patient to keep both eyes open while inserting the lens and allow adequate amount of time to the patient for the lens to settle down as much as possible on the eye prior to any lens fitting assessment.

FITTING ASSESSMENT

Usually patient takes 5–15 minutes to adapt. Check fit once the lens settles down. The optometrist needs to assess following:

Corneal Coverage

The overall lens diameter should allow the full coverage of the entire cornea. Full coverage implies that the lens should overlap the entire cornea at least by 1 mm in all position of gaze.

Assessment of corneal coverage is, therefore, done in all gazes. Inadequate corneal coverage implies the need of larger diameter or steeper base curve. If you alter the lens diameter, it will alter the sagittal value which alters the lens-cornea relationship. Therefore, it is mandatory to increase the BOZR, if you increase the total lens diameter. The guideline is "increase in total lens diameter by 0.50 mm demands an increase in BOZR by 0.30 mm".

Incomplete corneal coverage will result in irritations, watering, or corneal desiccation.

Lens Centration

Lens centration is very critical for good visual performance and comfortable wearing of the lenses. Ideally, lens edges should not rest on limbal area and patient should look through the optical zone of the lens. Decentrations of 0.2–0.75 mm in the primary gaze position are acceptable. Edge fitting and the BOZR are two critical factors to ensure good lens centration. Use diffuse illumination technique with slit lamp to observe lens centration.

Lens Movement

Lens movement removes and disperses debris from below the lens and is affected by host of factors which include lens design, lens type, lens material, and fitting philosophy. Lids have lot of potential to induce lens movement. Ideally, SCL should move with every blink. The ideal movement during blinking is taken as 0.50–1.00 mm. Movement more than this implies the need for steeper base curve or larger diameter and no movement implies flatter base curve or smaller diameter. Use diffuse illumination technique with slit lamp to assess postblink lens movement in primary gaze.

The lens movement should also be observed in different gaze position with slit lamp. Lateral gaze lag up to 1.5 mm and upgaze lag of 1.5 mm down imply well-fitting lens. Always avoid nonmoving lens which will result in accumulation of cellular debris behind the lens and excessively moving lens which will lead to potential corneal exposure and unstable vision (Fig. 3.1).

Lens Tightness

The lens tightness is assessed using "push up test" (Fig. 3.2). Hold the lower lid margin with your index finger and manipulate the lens position with the front lid margin to push up. A tight lens will be difficult to displace, whereas a loose lens will be easily displaced. A tight lens will also be sluggish to recenter. Lens tightness can also be assessed by postblink fluctuations in vision. A tight lens exhibits better vision immediately after blink, whereas a loose lens exhibits blur vision immediately after blink. Lens edge fitting and base curve

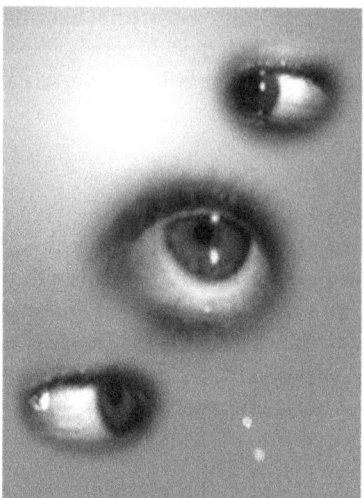

Fig. 3.1: Lens movement on different gaze.

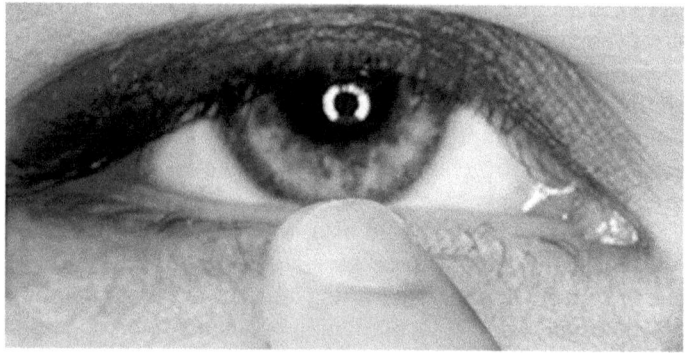

Fig. 3.2: Push up test.

of the lens are important fitting parameters for lens tightness. Lens edge curling or wrinkling are obvious signs of loose lens.

Comfort

A successful lens fitting implies that lens provides an increased comfort to the wearer. A lens that moves less may provide more subjective comfort to the wearer than the lens that moves more. Lid-lens interaction is also responsible for the wearing comfort of the lens. In case the patient reports discomfort, check for base curve and lens diameter.

> **Box 3.1:** TRAITS OF GOOD SOFT CONTACT LENS FIT.
> - Stable, clear, and consistent vision
> - Subjective comfort
> - Full corneal coverage
> - A good keratometric mire reflex with lens on the eye
> - Well-defined retinoscopy reflex
> - Ideal lens movement with perfect centration

Vision Stability

Assess the vision of the patient after 15–20 minutes of the lens insertion. A good lens fit will provide consistent and clear vision to the wearer. Perform over-refraction to detect the residual refractive error and to arrive at the correct lens power. A steeper or flatter lens fit will result in mismatch of over-refraction results with the spectacle refraction done earlier. Acceptance of excessive minus will be noticed in case of a steep lens fitting (Box 3.1).

Lens Delivery

Patient education as to lens wearing and maintenance is critical to the success of SCL fitting. A good fit lens will be used over a period of time only if the patient knows how to handle them, how to maintain them, and when to replace them. It is, therefore, very important for the practitioner to instruct them about insertion and removal techniques, educate him on lens handling and lens care, assure him about the normal adaptive symptoms like lens awareness, mild redness or dryness, prescribe suitable solution, recommend wearing schedule, advice replacement schedule, and finally insist on spare pair and follow-ups with him.

ALTERING SOFT CONTACT LENS PARAMETERS

Changing Total Lens Diameter

An increase in lens diameter will tighten the fit if all other factors remain unaltered. A decrease in diameter will loosen the fit. If the diameter is increased, the BOZR must also be increased to offset the effect the diameter change.

The thumb rule for SCL is an increase in diameter by 0.5 mm needs an increase in BOZR by 0.3 mm.

Example:
    BOZR = 8.6 mm, TD = 13.5 mm
    Desired TD = 14.0 mm

Final lens:
BOZR = 8.9 mm, TD = 14.0 mm

Changing Back Optic Zone Radius

A higher BOZR in mm flattens the lens and a lower BOZR steepens the lens fitting. Therefore, a compensatory adjustment must be made in TD of the lens to maintain the same lens-cornea relation. The thumb rule is if BOZR is increased by 0.3 mm, the TD must also be increased by 0.50 mm for the aforesaid purpose.

SOFT CONTACT LENS CARE SYSTEM

Inadequate or improper care of soft hydrogel lens may lead to ocular problems, patient discomfort, and ultimately drop out. The care system for SCL requires a wide range of antimicrobial care system which has to be nontoxic to the cornea and must fulfill following requirements:
- Kill microorganism
- Remove deposits
- Keep the lens hydrated
- Condition lens surface
- Maintain compatibility and wettability.

In order to achieve the aforesaid goals, the lens care system must comprise of the following components:
- Cleaning
- Rinsing
- Disinfecting
- Lubricating
- Deproteinizing
- Contact lens case cleaning.

Cleaning

The purpose of cleaning is to remove debris, deposits, cosmetics, and microorganisms. Lenses should be cleaned each time they are removed from the eyes. Rubbing both the sides of the lens with fingers is essential for cleaning.

Rinsing

Once the lenses are cleaned, they must be rinsed. Rinsing removes the loosened debris and ensures the solutions compatibility and tear pH at the time of insertion.

Disinfecting

Disinfection kills the microorganism and maintains the lens hydration. There are two types of disinfection procedure—heat-based procedure and chemical-based disinfection procedure. Heat-based disinfection procedure causes alterations within the lens. Chemical disinfection utilizes either preservatives or hydrogen peroxide to remove microorganism.

Lubricating

Lubricants are wetting agents. They decrease the wetting angle of the contact lens material. Poloxamine, hydroxypropyl methylcellulose, and tetronic 1304 are common.

Deproteinizing

Protein removers are another important component of lens care system, especially high water content ionic SCL and may be recommended on weekly basis as an additional lens care procedure. Enzyme-based cleaners are available in tablet form which is dissolved in multipurpose solution (MPS) and the lens is kept for 15 minutes to 2 hours in the solution. Papain, subtilisin, pronase, and pancreatin are enzymes.

Contact Lens Case Cleaning

Contact lenses must be stored in a clean lens case. A soiled case can be the cause of ocular infection when contaminants are transferred to a contact lens and from the lens to the eye. It can also be the cause of lens discoloration. If a lens case is heavily contaminated with microorganisms, it may reduce the efficacy of the disinfection system. The lens case should be rinsed after every use and the lenses should be stored in fresh solution. In addition, the following steps may be followed on regular interval:
- Discard all used solutions from the case.
- Scrub the lens case with toothbrush and detergent or oil-free soaps weekly.
- Rinse the case with warm water and rub thoroughly with clean, dry tissue.
- Air dry the case. A dry case will prevent colonization by microorganisms.
- It is prudent to replace the lens case at frequent intervals.

There were three bottles care system, but today almost all the disinfection system are in the form of MPS—one bottle solution. These MPSs contain complex combination of ingredients. Surfactants in the form of borate and citrate are present in low amounts in MPS, whereas they are in higher concentration in separately packaged cleaners. They remove mucin, debris, contaminants, and eye make up to help maintain a clean and wettable lens surface. Alcohol-based cleaners are good at dissolving lipids. Buffering agents keep the pH of the solution close to the natural tears and are included in the rinsing solution. They also aid in cleaning and disinfection. Sodium borate and boric acid are common buffering agents. They also form an essential ingredient of the MPS. Preservatives are antimicrobial agents such as polyaminopropyl biguanide, polyhexanide hydrochloride, and polyquaternium. First generation preservatives such as thimerosal or chlorhexidines or benzalkonium chloride have been found to create cytotoxic reactions. Some sensitive patients can still develop toxic reactions to preservatives. In addition to above, MPS also contains edetate disodium (EDTA) that prevents calcium bound proteins from depositing on the lens surface which also enhances disinfecting ability of the solution. Today, MPS represents the most popular mode of disinfection. They usually allow storage for up to 30 days in an unopened case without needing to change the solution.

Hydrogen peroxide based system is very effective chemical disinfection system for SCLs. The system is able to kill large number of microorganism in a short period of time. On an average, 10-15 minutes is enough for complete disinfection of lenses. However, direct contact with the solution causes ocular discomfort. Hence, the solution must be neutralized prior to reinsertion of the lens into the eyes. Once the system is neutralized, it loses its antimicrobial power. Only water, sodium chloride, and stabilizer remain. Neutralization may be completed in single step or two steps. In case of single step neutralization, platinum disk is used as catalytic for neutralization. A vented lens case is taken to allow oxygen generated to escape and the lens with the tablet is put into the solution. After a recommended period of time which may extend up to 6 hours, lenses can be reinserted into the eyes.

In case of two step system, neutralization is performed as a separate step or another solution is required for neutralization. The biggest advantage of this method is that time taken for disinfecting can vary and therefore, suitable for occasional wearer. But this is an expensive procedure.

If the SCL is dropped while insertion, the wearer should be advised to rinse the lens with sterile saline solution without rubbing.

FITTING SILICONE HYDROGEL LENSES

The new family of silicone hydrogel soft lenses usually termed as "superpermeable" contact lenses can transmit unprecedented amount of oxygen to the cornea. The main difficulty with silicone material is that its natural surface is extremely hydrophobic which means the surface wettability is extremely poor, causing excessive lipid deposition. Another big issue is extremely low water content of the material which means the fluid is unable to flow through these lens material, resulting in frequent lens binding to the ocular surface. In traditional hydrogel lenses, the polyHEMA itself is not oxygen permeable, so the water performs the job of carrying oxygen through the lens to the cornea. Silicone material itself is highly oxygen permeable. Silicone hydrogel lens material is a combination of silicone rubber and hydrogel polymer.

The ideal fitting method for silicone hydrogel lenses should be similar to that of any well fit hydrogel lenses. However, while fitting silicone hydrogel lenses, the practitioner should keep following things in his mind:

- Patient may experience a high level of initial awareness with silicone hydrogel lenses because of higher modulus of elasticity. The higher modulus of material lessens the degree to which the lens flexes and conforms itself to the corneal surface, as compared to the standard hydrogel lenses. Therefore, the relationship between the lens and the corneal surface must be more precise.
- Silicone hydrogel lenses may display a tendency to "flute" at the edge, if the lens-to-cornea relationship is not correct.
- Different silicone hydrogel material has different water content and different Dk value, resulting in different modulus of elasticity. Increase in water content reduces modulus and at the same time ensures good lens movement, but it reduces Dk/t. On the other hand, increased silicone rubber increases Dk but makes the lens stiffer and easy to handle. In order to appreciate the importance of oxygen performance of a contact lens, it is necessary to understand how much oxygen the cornea requires to maintain normal physiology. The best known criteria have been proposed by Holden and Mertz who stated that in order to achieve no corneal swelling during daily wear, an oxygen transmissibility of 24.1 units

is required. They also proposed that during overnight wear, a lens with a minimum Dk/t of 87 units is required. However, neither of this value is edge corrected and when this correction is applied the values becomes 21. 8 and 73, respectively.

There is a need for good in depth counseling as to the material's rigidity, its initial feel, and perceived comfort for a successful fit and may also be an important variable in selecting the appropriate candidate, particularly when a candidate is switching over from traditional hydrogel lenses. Once this is done, a complete routine procedure with particular emphasis upon following factors has to be completed:

Base Curve Selection

Taking keratometer readings are important, as standard 8.6 mm may not be ideal choice in all cases. In certain cases, edge fluting may be seen which can be solved if the base curve is changed to 8.4 mm. As a general rule, silicone hydrogel lenses are fitted on the steeper side to distribute the weight of the lens evenly because of its high modulus.

Movement Test

On primary gaze, the lens should move between 0.2 mm and 0.5 mm and on superior gaze up to 0.8 mm. The tightness of the lens may be assessed by "push up test". In general, silicone hydrogel lens tends to move more than the conventional hydrogel lenses, giving an impression that the lens is loose. Fitting should allow adequate tear exchange for debris and bacteria removal.

Trial Method

Empirical method of fitting the lens is not recommended for silicone hydrogel lenses. Trial lens method is the most ideal method. Trial must be done with lens material to be dispensed, not with any other material. Lid scrubbing with Johnson and Johnson baby shampoo is recommended before putting the first trial lens in the eye to remove oil from meibomian glands.

Dispense the Lens

When you remove the trial lens from the patient's eyes, ask him to blink several times; mucin balls, if any, will go away. Silicone hydrogel lenses should be dispensed as "lens and prescribed solution package". Hydrogen peroxide system of lens care system works better for silicone hydrogel lenses. Hydrogen peroxide penetrates the lens material providing thorough cleaning and removing microbes. It is also able to break proteins and lipid bond and remove trapped debris. In addition, it can penetrate microbial biofilm, which most of the MPS cannot do. It is also preservative free—ideal for patients who have hypersensitivities or dry eyes. The solution must be neutralized before placing lens on to the eyes. The idea of "no rub" may work to remove loosely bound, nondenatured proteins that are found on conventional hydrogel lenses. Silicone hydrogel lenses deposit small amount of denatured proteins and increased amount of lipid; therefore, the patient using silicone hydrogel lens should rub the lenses with their prescribed MPS if they are to maintain optical performance. However, if lipid deposits are not been removed by rubbing with MPS, adding surfactant cleaners may work. In addition, lid hygiene care regimen should be prescribed to remove oil from meibomian glands, cleaning the lid margins with Ciba's eye scrub, or Johnson and Johnson baby shampoo to remove oil from meibomian glands. Finally, the lens should be delivered with a comprehensive advice for follow up program. Every patient who begins on overnight wear should be seen on the following morning. The daily wearer should be asked to visit on the 1st week, 1st month, 3rd month, and then every 6 month after dispensing the lens.

Silicone Hydrogel Lens Care System

The silicone hydrogel lens material is different from that of hydrogel lens material. A comparison between two tells us that:
- Silicone material in its natural surface is extremely hydrophobic, which means the surface wettability is extremely poor as compare to hydrogel lens material.
- They deposit lipids more readily than the hydrogel material. Protein deposits are less.
- Another big issue is extremely low water content of the material which means the fluid is unable to flow through these lens material, resulting in frequent lens binding to the ocular surface.
- The material modulus of elasticity is higher than the soft hydrogel lenses which increases material stiffness.

Hydrophobicity and lipid attraction implies that mechanical rubbing is very critical to clean the lens surface. MiraFlow is alcohol-based daily cleaner and can emulsify lipids as well as provide some lens disinfection. AOSept by CIBA for disinfection, MiraFlow as daily cleaner, and the third bottle, Softwear saline, needed to rinse off the MiraFlow prior to disinfection, is the good care regimen.

FITTING DISPOSABLE SOFT CONTACT LENSES

In the recent years, the concept of early lens replacement has become popular. Now, people think of replacing their old lens quite often to ensure healthy and fresh vision. Accordingly, lenses have been developed to have planned replacement program. The lenses which are disposed off every day with another lens is termed as daily disposable and the lenses that are disposed off every month with a new one are put into the category of monthly disposable lenses. Basically, these lenses are thinner and high water content than the conventional soft lenses. They do not require use of protein removing tablets, and in fact, daily disposable lenses do not require any lens care system. The ideal fitting method for disposable soft lenses should be similar to that of any well fit soft lenses.

SOFT CONTACT LENS FITTING IN DRY EYES

The main objective of lens fitting in patients with dry eyes is to reduce the effects of evaporation and pervaporation. Soft hydrogel contact lenses are not the right choice. In case they are fitted, the following guideline should be followed:
- Try ionic material, if replaced frequently. Otherwise nonionic material
- Thicker lens
- Low water content
- Minimal wearing schedule
- Unpreserved lubricants
- Preservative-free lens care products.

Frequent replacements reduces the front surface deposits that disrupts tear film and lead to shorter BUT.

INSTRUCTIONS FOR SOFT LENS INSERTION

- Put the wet and clean right lens on the tip of the index finger or middle finger of your dominant hand.
- Ensure that the lens is correct side out. The edges should face upward (bowl shape), and not outward (saucer shape).
- Or, one can do the TACO test. Place the lens over the heart line of your palm and fold your palm gradually and gently. If the lens is correct side out, both the edges will come together. If not, the edges will move away from each other, toward the palm.

- Now pull down the lower lid with the middle or ring finger of the same hand. Use your other hand to hold the upper lid together with lashes; open the eye firmly.
- Look directly at the lens or into a mirror and place the lens directly on cornea.
- Release your lower lid first and then slowly release your upper lid.
- Close the eye and massage with index finger from top of the eyelids to position the lens.
- Repeat the procedure for your other eye.

INSTRUCTIONS FOR SOFT LENS REMOVAL

- Look up and pull the lower lid down with the middle finger of your dominant hand.
- Place your index finger on the lower edge of your lens and slide the lens down to the white of your eye.
- Squeeze the lens lightly between your index finger and thumb and remove gently.
- Repeat the procedure for the other eye.

MULTIPLE CHOICE QUESTIONS

Q. 1. The HVID of a patient is 11.80 mm; suggest the appropriate total lens diameter of the initial SCL for the patient.
   a. 13.80 mm
   b. 13.50 mm
   c. 14.50 mm
   d. 14.00 mm

Q. 2. When considering the BOZR selection of the initial trial lens while fitting soft contact lenses, which of the following statement seems to be true?
   a. Add 0.80 mm to the flatter K-reading
   b. Add 1.00 mm to the average K-reading
   c. BOZR is relatively unimportant for very thin soft contact lenses but is very important for thicker soft contact lenses
   d. All of the above

ANSWERS

| 1. a | 2. d |

Q. 3. Which of the following statement is important to consider while considering the total lens diameter of soft contact lens for a patient?
a. Increase in total lens diameter by 0.50 mm demands an increase in BOZR by 0.30 mm
b. Increase in total lens diameter by 0.50 mm demands a decrease in BOZR by 0.30 mm
c. Increase in total lens diameter by 0.50 mm demands an increase in BOZR by 0.50 mm
d. Increase in total lens diameter by 0.50 mm demands a decrease in BOZR by 0.30 mm

Q. 4. A soft contact lens wearer complains that his vision clears for short while just immediately after a blink. What could be the possible cause?
a. The fitting of the lens is too tight
b. The fitting of the lens is too flat
c. The lens shows excess movement on eye
d. The BOZR of the lens is too small

Q. 5. An SCL wearer complains that his vision blurs immediately after a blink and then quickly comes back to previous clear vision. What could be the possible cause?
a. The fitting of the lens is too tight
b. The fitting of the lens is too flat
c. The BVP of the lens is not correctly given
d. The patient is malingering

Q. 6. Which of the following shows the signs of a tight soft lens fitting?
a. A tightly fit SCL will be difficult to displace during the push up test
b. A tightly fit soft lens will be sluggish to recenter
c. A tight lens exhibits improved vision immediately after blink
d. All of the above

Q. 7. Which of the following explains the ideal fit of SCLs?
a. The lens edge should not rest on the limbal area
b. The SCL should overlap the entire cornea at least by 1 mm in all gaze direction
c. The lens should move at least 0.50–1.00 mm with each blink
d. All of the above

ANSWERS

3. a   4. a   5. b   6. d   7. d

Q. 8. Which of the following is not the characteristic of a good soft contact lens fitting?
  a. Lens edge curling or wrinkling
  b. Lens moves with every blink
  c. Well-defined retinoscopy reflex
  d. A good keratometric mire reflex with the lens on the eye

Q. 9. Why is rinsing an important function of soft contact lens care and maintenance?
  a. Rinsing removes residual cleaners
  b. Rinsing rehydrates the lens
  c. Rinsing removes the loosened lens contaminants
  d. All of the above

Q. 10. While assessing SCL fitting, ideal lens movement in primary gaze during blinking is:
  a. 1–1.5 mm
  b. 0.8–1.5 mm
  c. 0.5–1 mm
  d. 0.75–1.5 mm

Q. 11. In order to check for ideal SCL fitting on eye, which of the following elements are important to check?
  a. Corneal coverage and lens centration
  b. Lens movement and lens tightness
  c. Comfort and vision stability
  d. All of the above

Q.12. If contact lens user complains of dryness symptoms at end of the day, which of the following examination is not needed?
  a. Lid examination
  b. Dryness test
  c. Duochrome test
  d. Contact lens fitting assessment

ANSWERS

| 8. a | 9. d | 10. c | 11. d | 12. c |

Chapter 4

Fitting Soft Toric Lenses

INTRODUCTION

The use of soft toric lenses in preference to spherical soft lens is indicated when the ocular astigmatism is present—be it corneal or otherwise that warrants correction. Astigmatism is an optical defect, whereby vision is blurred due to the inability of the optics of the eye to focus a point object into a sharp point image on the retina. Literally, the optical system of the eye does not form a point image. This may be due to irregular or toric curvature of the cornea or the lens:
- There may be meridional differences in curvature of the cornea and crystalline lens.
- The shape of the posterior pole of crystalline lens may be toric in shape, or it may be tilted.

Unlike rigid lens, spherical soft lens do not mask corneal astigmatism, instead conform to the shape of the cornea. Consequently, correcting ocular astigmatism with soft lenses requires that cylinder be incorporated into back vertex power (BVP) of the lens.

INDICATIONS

In order to decide whether to fit or not to fit a toric soft lens, practitioners should assess each patient individually and should not be guided by any established criteria such as "all patients with cylinder greater than a certain amount should be fitted with soft toric lenses". In general, toric soft lenses are found to be lenses of choice in the following cases:
- As a general rule, 0.75 D or more of astigmatism should be corrected.
- When best sphere does not give satisfactory visual acuity.
- If the astigmatism is lenticular or party noncorneal, toric soft lens are better option than spherical rigid gas permeable (RGP) lens.
- Patients who are not able to adapt to RGP lenses.
- When the sphere to cylinder ratio is less than 4:1.

- ATR astigmatism is more suitable for toric soft contact lens (SCL). However, care must be taken to rule out following cases:
- Patients with low spherical component are less likely to be successful with toric SCL (e.g. +0.25/-2.75 × 180°).
- Oblique cylinder will have poor lens stability due to lens-lid interaction (e.g. -1.50/-1.50 × 45°).
- The larger cylinder necessitates greater accuracy as degree of rotation becomes important with high cylinder (+3.00/-6.00 × 80°).
- If lens rotation is more than 25° or compensation by more than 20° is needed, it implies that new lens will have different fitting than what is being observed during trial.

CLASSIFICATION OF ASTIGMATISM (TABLE 4.1)

TABLE 4.1: Classification of astigmatism.

Corneal astigmatism	• It occurs when the front curve of the cornea is irregularly shaped • It can be measured by keratometer
Lenticular astigmatism	• It occurs because of meridional difference in the refractive power of crystalline lens • A tilted or decentered lens may also induce lenticular astigmatism
Internal astigmatism	• The posterior pole inside the eye may be toric in shape or tilted leading to internal astigmatism
Total astigmatism	• Summation of corneal, lental, and internal astigmatism • It can be measured by retinoscopy and subjective refraction
With-the-rule astigmatism	• Refractive power of vertical meridian is greater and the axis is located horizontally
Against-the-rule astigmatism	• Refractive power of horizontal meridian is greater and the axis is located vertically
Oblique astigmatism	• Two axis lies somewhere between the axes defining either WTR or ATR
Regular astigmatism	• Regular astigmatism is the type of astigmatism where principal meridian are 90° apart
Irregular astigmatism	• Irregular astigmatism is the type of astigmatism where principal meridian are not 90° apart • Irregular astigmatism is mostly the result of trauma or disease
Residual astigmatism	• Astigmatism that remains uncorrected when contact lenses are placed upon the cornea to correct the existing refractive error

(ATR: Against-the-rule; WTR: With-the-rule)

FITTING METHODS

In case of toric lens, lens rotation and stability on the eye is the additional important issue which has to be understood and is perhaps the most frustrating aspect of fitting toric lenses. The reason is fairly simple—astigmatic correction depends a lot on a stable and centered lens.

Toric lenses can be fitted empirically or by trial lens fitting. Under empirical fitting method, lenses are ordered based on the patient's spectacle refraction, corneal curvature, and lens diameter as measured. The patient does not get the feel of the lens before the final lens is delivered to him. The lenses fitted empirically are usually fitted on manufacturer's recommendations and do not rotate on the eyes.

Not all patients can be fitted with soft toric lenses empirically. Some practitioner also uses diagnostic lens to fit toric lenses. Trial lenses made in toric lens design but without cylinder incorporation is manufactured which are chosen based on back optic zone radius (BOZR) and spherocylinder over refraction is performed. Lens orientation and fitting is assessed before the lens is ordered.

However, the most common method used for trial lens fitting is the use of toric trial lenses which also incorporates the cylinder correction. The sequential step-by-step procedure is as under:

- *Step 1:* Complete subjective refraction and note down the spectacle prescription in minus cylinder form, e.g. -6.00/-1.75 × 180°.
- *Step 2:* Next, keratometry is to be done to find the corneal curvature of two principal meridians. Add 0.80 mm to flattest meridian. Flattest meridian is the larger reading in mm or smaller reading in diopter.
- *Step 3:* Compensate the spectacle prescription for vertex distance (Fig. 4.1). Each meridian values should be compensated separately. For example, spectacle refraction is -6.00/-1.75 × 180°
- *Step 4:* Select a toric trial lens as close to the results of step 3 and put the lenses on the patient's eyes.
- *Step 5:* Allow 15-20 minutes time for the lens to settle, orient, and be adapted.
- *Step 6:* Assess the complete aspects of lens fitting including lens coverage, centration, movement, and the comfort.
- *Step 7:* Assess rotational behavior.
- *Step 8:* Compensate for lens rotation and apply LARS (left add, right subtract) or CASS (clockwise add, anti-clockwise subtract).
- *Step 9:* Design final lens power and order.

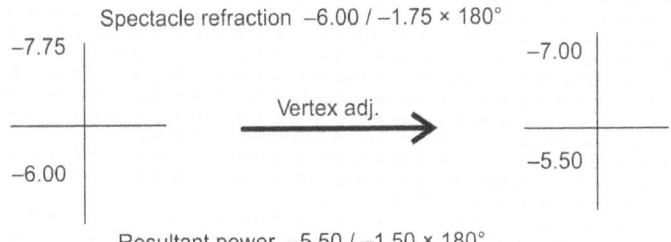

Fig. 4.1: Vertex calculations in toric lens fitting.

It is important to remember that one must avoid over-refraction while fitting toric soft lenses under this method.

ROTATIONAL BEHAVIOR

Probably, the most important factor while fitting soft toric lens is their orientation on the eye which is determined by their rotational behavior. On average, toric soft contact lenses will tend to rotate nasally or anticlockwise by about 5–10°. Nasal rotation is the rotation toward the nose with respect to the inferior aspect or base of the lens. However, the actual magnitude and direction of lens rotation is subject to large individual variations and depends on lot of factors. In order to facilitate the assessment of rotational behavior of the lens, all soft toric lenses available have some sort of reference mark which helps to assess the dynamics of orientation of the soft toric lens. These reference markings are extremely important as they form the basis of the lens prescription. Unless the orientation is measured and assessed quantitatively and qualitatively, the perfect toric lens prescription cannot be decided accurately. These reference markings are usually located a short distance from the lens edge at 6 O'clock, 3 O'clock, and 9 O'clock or 12 O'clock or in three positions (Fig. 4.2). The manufacturer usually place a reference mark or marks on the lens so that its rotational behavior can be assessed when the lens is on the eye. This reference marking does not represent the cylinder axis. These may be in the form of ink or photochemical dots, laser marks, scribe lines, or engraved dots.

Lens mislocation is measured as the deviation from the vertical, if the markings are located at 6 or 12 O'clock or from the horizontal if the markings are located at 3 and 9 O'clock position. The magnitude

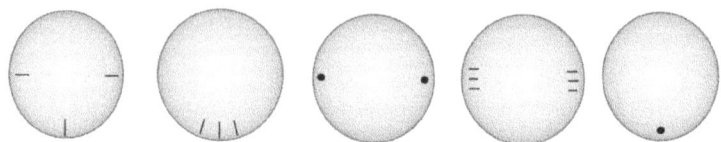

Fig. 4.2: Toric orientation laser marks.

and the direction of any deviation must be determined and used to compensate the ocular astigmatic axis mislocation.

MEASURING LENS ROTATION

Orientation of the soft toric lens has to be done quantitatively and qualitatively both. Quantitative assessment requires the assessment of any rotation and orientation position, and qualitative assessment requires assessment of rotational stability. But before measuring lens rotation:
- Assess physical fit of the lens.
- Be aware of the lens decentration.
- Full corneal coverage.
- Adequate movement in push up test and postblink movement test.
- Allow enough time for lens stabilization. Normally, 5-10 minutes are good enough for a perfectly fit lens to stabilize.

Quantitative measurement can be done by measuring rotation of the lens and its directional orientation is the key to successful soft toric lens fitting. Rotation has to be assessed with the blink and in different position of the gaze. The following methods may be applied:
- Use low cylinder trial lens.
- Put trial frame on the patient's eye.
- General lighting condition in the room.
- Use low cylindrical lens and align its axis with the contact lens reference mark, which gives the rotation of the toric lens.

Slit lamp can also be used to measure the lens rotation as under:
- Use of the rotating slit beam on the slit lamp.
- Majority of the slit lamp have protractor scale to determine the angle of the slit beam.
- With the illumination arm located centrally and a narrow slit selected, the slit is aligned with the reference mark on the lens.
- The angle of rotation can be read from the slit's protractor scale.

In some slit lamps, special purpose protractor scale eyepiece graticules is attached which can be used to measure toric lens rotation. The scale, which is in one eyepiece only, can be left in place during normal slit lamp use. The orientation of the reference marks can be read directly while observing the lens in the eye. This is perhaps the most accurate and direct method.

Besides, quantitative measurement, qualitative assessment is equally important to assess the following:
- Minimum rotation with blink
- Speed of reorientation.

COMPENSATING FOR THE LENS ROTATION

The final cylinder axis of the lens to be prescribed is determined by compensating the spectacle prescription axis to the rotational behavior of the trial lens. It is assumed that any subsequent lenses of the same design will exhibit identical behavior as that of the trial lens.

If the location marks are reliable and stable, the practitioner should note their position in relation to their intended position and the direction and degree of rotation seen, if any. The axis rotation gives the practitioner the information needed to order the next lens. The rotation of the lens shows how far the axis of the cylinder will be mislocated when the final lens is placed on the eye. Ordering a lens with the axis at a different position can compensate for this mislocation.

The following steps have to be followed:
- Evaluate rotation of the marks on the eye—whether it is clockwise or anticlockwise.
- Estimate degree of rotation as explained above—1 hour implies 30°.
- Apply LARS principle or CAAS principle.

The basic rule is that if the lens rotates clockwise, the degree of rotation should be added to the axis, but if the lens rotates anticlockwise the rotation should be subtracted from the axis (CAAS).

Alternatively, if the lens rotates to the left, the rotation should be added and if it is to the right it should be subtracted (LARS).

The rotation has to be assessed to the right or left of the practitioner and not the patient.

Example:
- Ocular refraction is $-2.00/-1.25 \times 180°$
- Trial lens rotates by 10° when placed on the eye to the left side of the practitioner.

- The correction acting on the eye now would be -2.00/-1.25 × 170°. The result: vision will be blurred.
- Compensating the rotation will result in the prescription: -2.00/-1.25×10°.
- 10° axis on rotation will bring the axis round to 180°, the required axis.

SELECTING A TORIC STABILIZATION DESIGN

In order to neutralize astigmatic refractive error effective, a toric lens aligns its axis of cylinder correction to the axis of astigmatic error. There are different stabilization designs that the lens manufacturer use to increase the lens stability so that the cylinder axis of the contact lens is aligned with the axis of astigmatic error of the patient. Some of the commonly used techniques are as under:

Prism Ballast

Prism ballast design employs 1-1.5 prism dioptre base down prism with maximum of 3 prism Diopter, with heaviest portion of the lens lying at 6 O'clock position below the lower lid. Gravitational forces help preventing lens rotation. Theoretically, it may induce vertical prismatic imbalance if used in one eye. The thicker portion also reduces oxygen transmissibility and some patient may feel discomfort along the lower lid margin caused by increased thickness of prism base (Fig. 4.3).

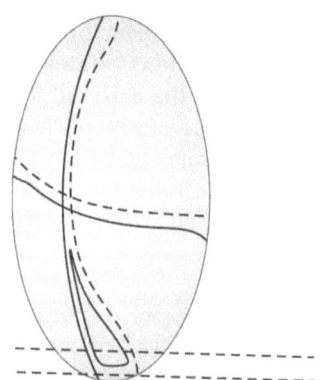

Fig. 4.3: Prism ballast.

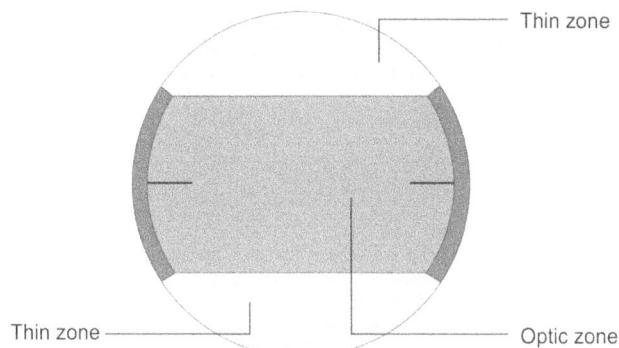

Fig. 4.4: Double slab off stabilization design.

Double Slab Off Stabilization Design

In double slab off stabilization design, the top and bottom of the lenses are chamfered to reduce the thickness for lens stabilization (Fig. 4.4). The squeezing pressure exerted by the upper eyelid provides the majority effect with lower eyelid assisting in stabilizing the lens. The central body lies along the palpebral fissure and thinner zones along the inferior and superior edges which come to lie under the upper and lower lids. The thickness of the lens plays an important role in stabilizing the lens rotation.

Accelerated Stability Design

Accelerated stability design has been created with the understanding of the eye dynamics and application of advanced manufacturing techniques. It has four stability zones and uses the force of the blink to stabilize the lens. When the lens is correctly aligned, minimal lid interaction happens. The upper and lower lid forces therefore continually orient and stabilize the lens to return to its correctly oriented position (Fig. 4.5).

The 8/4 Precision Balance Design

The 8/4 Precision Balance Design is the enhancement over prism ballast design. The thickest portions of the lens are located at 8 O'clock and 4 O'clock position, thus the thickness is divided into two positions. The superior portion of the lens is thinned to produce prism-like rotational stabilization effect. Diagonal forces of thicker area at 8 O'clock and 4 O'clock positions reduce lens rotation. The main advantages of this

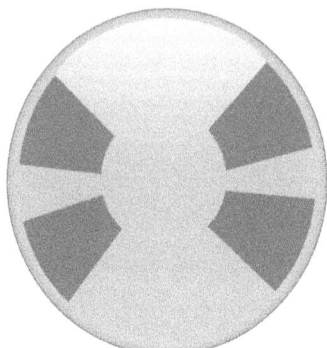

Fig. 4.5: Accelerated stability design.

technique are prism free optical design and reduced lens-lid interaction at lower lid margin that enhances comfort (Fig. 4.6).

While selecting a stabilization design for a patient, the practitioner should consider all those factors that would influence the lens behavior in the eye. Notable among them are:
- Position of lower lid
- Lid angles, whether sloping upward or downward
- Size of vertical palpebral aperture
- Lid tension
- Force and direction of movement on blink
- Lifestyle, for example dancers are more benefitted by nonprism ballast design.

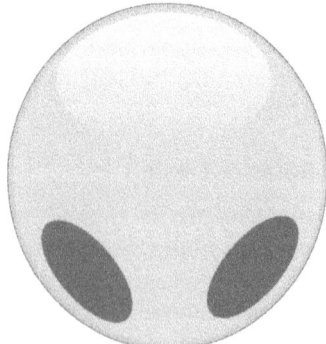

Fig. 4.6: The 8/4 precision balance design.

OVERREFRACTION

Overrefraction in case of toric lens trial is a challenging affair. However, if the lens rotation is within 10° of its desired position, overrefraction may be conducted with spherical trial lens to decide the final spherical component. A lens that rotates will yield residual astigmatism, indicating the poor stabilization of the lens.

> **IMPORTANT POINTS TO REMEMBER**
> - If the rotation is more than 30°, do not fit the same lens. Try alternate design.
> - Maximum amount of axis rotation acceptable is 10°.
> - Fluctuating vision through a toric soft lens is usually attributed to poor rotation stability.
> - If the lens rotates excessively, consider steepening the lens fit or increase the overall diameter of the lens or select a different lens design.
> - Compensation for more than 20° or more means that new lens will be quite different to that trialed and the outcome is unlikely to be as expected.

MULTIPLE CHOICE QUESTIONS

Q. 1. Which of the following is the correct answer to indicate for soft toric contact lenses fitting?
  a. When astigmatism is 0.75 D or more
  b. When best sphere does not give satisfactory visual acuity
  c. If the astigmatism is lenticular or partly noncorneal
  d. All of the above

Q. 2. Which of the following is the most likely to be successful with soft toric contact lenses?
  a. −2.00/−1.25 @180   b. −1.50/−1.50 @45
  c. +3.00/−6.00 @80   d. +0.25/−3.00 @180

Q. 3. A toric soft contact lens has BVP of −2.25/−2.50 @135. Which of the following meridian will have greatest thickness?
  a. 135° meridian   b. 45° meridian
  c. 55° meridian   d. 145° meridian

ANSWERS

| 1. d | 2. a | 3. b |

Q. 4. What does the reference mark on soft toric lens denote?
   a. Lens orientation in situ
   b. Axis of cylinder
   c. Standard stabilization location
   d. Reference to hold the lens while wearing and removing

Q. 5. Which of the following statement is not correct for soft toric lenses fitting?
   a. The rotation of soft toric lens should be minimum.
   b. The rotation of soft toric lens has to be assessed to the right or left of the patient.
   c. Fluctuating vision through a soft toric lens is usually attributed to poor rotational stability.
   d. If the soft toric lens rotates excessively, consider steepening the lens fit.

Answers

| 4. a | 5. b |

CHAPTER 5

Spherical RGP Lens Fitting

INTRODUCTION

One of the most important reasons for fitting rigid gas permeable (RGP) lenses is the desire to have good visual acuity and no ocular insult. If fitted properly, the patient enjoys better visual performance than the soft contact lenses. Fitting RGP lenses takes more chair time. A good and dynamic approach to fit RGP lens is to try two different diameter in two eyes as in almost all cases the two eyes requires same total diameter.

INDICATIONS

Motivation is a key factor in RGP lens fitting as initial adaptation period is relatively larger during which the wearer needs to tolerate the lens. A highly motivated potential wearer is likely to be more successful. Potential wearer with moderate-to-high prescription tends to be more motivated than those with lower power requirement. This may be possibly due to their unaided visual acuity as they cannot function without some sort of visual correction and they also carry a strong desire to get rid of their thick and heavy glasses.

The general rule is that the patients, who require an astigmatic visual correction, are better suited to RGP lens because of superior quality of vision as compared to soft lenses. The correction of high corneal astigmatism error, often defined as 2.50 D or greater, is best managed by either a back surface toric or bitoric RGP lenses. If a spherical RGP lens is fitted to a highly toric cornea, poor alignment of lens to cornea is present.

FITTING METHODS

The fitting of RGP lenses have to be more precise to the shape of the cornea because unlike soft lenses they do not drape over the corneal surface. Studies have shown that quality of RGP lens fit, if done purely empirically, is not as satisfactory as it is with trial lens fitting. Fluorescein pattern evaluation has been critical and crucial to evaluate the fit of RGP contact lenses. Fluorescein sodium either in the form of strip or in the form of dye is used to observe the tear film thickness between the lens and the cornea. The preferred method of instilling fluorescein sodium into the eye is to use a filter strip impregnated with the dye. A drop of nonpreserved saline is placed on the orange (impregnated) tip of fluorescein strip. The patient is instructed to look down and the strip is lightly touched on the superior conjunctiva for less than 1 second. The patient is instructed to execute a couple of blinks in order to spread the fluorescein. Placing a drop of fluorescein on the superior sclera will maximize the length of time the dye remains in the eye.

INITIAL DATA GATHERING

The best philosophy to be followed for fitting RGP lens should be "first trial lens placed on the patient's eye guide to the final fit". The following general guideline is recommended based on this philosophy:
- Lens total diameter selection
- Initial base curve selection
- Initial lens power selection.

Lens Total Diameter Selection

Since it is difficult to define the corneal periphery, the horizontal visible iris diameter (HVID) is used as a guide to the corneal diameter. The thumb rule for initial lens diameter is 2 mm smaller than the HVID measurement. The selection of total lens diameter is also influenced by the additional factors given in Table 5.1.

BOZD is decided by measuring the pupil diameter in dim light plus 1 mm.

Initial Base Curve Selection

The initial selection of base curve is adjusted with respect to the keratometric readings, which give the curvature of the corneal cap or apex. With regard to the K reading, K usually refers to the flatter of the two reading taken. For example, with readings of 45.00 D at 180° and 42.00 D at 90°, 42.00 D would be flatter reading and would be the value of K for the selection of initial trial lens for RGP fitting. This is typically related to the amount of corneal cylinder present.

Spherical RGP Lens Fitting

TABLE 5.1: Factors affecting total lens diameter.

Factors	Points to consider
Palpebral aperture size	A patient with a wide palpebral aperture is more likely to need a larger lens diameter, e.g. 10.00 mm or 10.50 mm. This helps the upper lid grasp the lens edge to prevent the lens riding low
Lid tonicity	If the lids are loose then, typically, a larger lens diameter is needed to provide optimum performance
Base curve	The flatter the cornea, the larger the lens diameter. An approximate table may be designed as under:

Base curve in diopter	Lens diameter
40.00–43.00 D	9.40 mm
43.25–45.00 D	9.20 mm
Greater than 45.00 D	9.00 mm

Another class of practitioners is of opinion that the base curve of the initial trial lens for spherical RGP lens should be selected slightly steeper than the flattest meridian. Now the question of how much steeper is answered by taking the mean of the two keratometer readings.

Lens Power Selection

The power of the initial RGP trial lens is selected as under:
- Convert the manifest refraction or the spectacle correction to minus cylinder form. For example, 7.00 Dsph + 1.50 Dcyl × 180° transposes to –6.00 Dsph –1.50 Dcyl × 90°.
- Drop the cylinder power and use only the spherical component of the prescription. In our example, it becomes –6.00 Dsph.
- Adjust for vertex correction to zero. In our above example, –6.00 Dsph at 12 mm vertex to a zero becomes –5.62 Dsph
- Select the lens power which is nearest to –5.62 Dsph in our trial lens. In case of +6.00 Dsph, the power would have been adjusted to +6.50 Dsph.
- Select the lens from the trial set within ± 4.00 D. If the power difference is more, then, it is always possible to have mismatch in the final lens fitting as compared to trial lens fitting. This is especially important in plus power where gravitational effects on the lens design is significant and in minus power there may be a difference in lens-lid relation due to edge difference.
- The cylindrical element dropped will be taken care of by the "tear lens".

TRIAL LENS SELECTION

Once the initial data has been gathered, the first trial lens should be selected in such a way so that it may guide us to the final lens fit. However, before inserting the trial lens into the patient's eyes, the practitioner must counsel the patient on the sensation they will notice when the lens will be placed on the cornea. The care must be taken while describing the sensation that the patient is not going to be alarmed. Advise them to keep their eyes shut for the first few minutes after the lens insertion and then maintain inferior direction of gaze when they begin to blink. Primary and upward gaze causes excessive discomfort, irritation, and tearing. An adequate amount of time must be allowed to the patient for the lens to settle down as much as possible on the eye prior to any lens fitting assessment.

FITTING ASSESSMENT

The lens fit is, then, assessed. Dynamic and static fitting of each lens trialed must be analyzed to achieve the optimum fitting for the patient.

Dynamic Fit

The dynamic aspects of the fitting are first observed with the eye in primary gaze and blinking normally. Observation can be made with the slit lamp which provides illumination and magnification.

The slit lamp may be employed with diffuse illumination to view the lens dynamic fitting characteristics. The patient may be asked to alter the direction of gaze to enable the practitioner to observe a better understanding of the nature of dynamic fitting.

The following aspects of the fitting are important:
- Assess the lens decentration, i.e. the location of the lens on the cornea. RGP lenses are rarely perfectly centered on the cornea. The decentration of the lens is determined by comparing the geometric center of the cornea with that of the lens. It may be done both in horizontal and vertical meridians. Excessive decentration may cause poor visual performance and lens instability resulting in discomfort. A steep lens on cornea is always more stable.
- The lens movement is initiated by the lid action and hence the assessment of lens movement on the cornea is an important factor while analyzing the lens fit. The lens moves down and up with the lid and then recenters to its position. Postblink recentration is important factor while analyzing the lens fit on the cornea.

Box 5.1: Traits of ideal dynamic fitting of rigid gas permeable (RGP) lens.

- Well-centered (±0.50 mm)
- Well-stable lens
- Smooth vertical movement at an average speed
- Lens rests uniformly across the corneal surface, ensuring good tear exchange
- Consistent lens movement will be seen with the change in position of eye gaze

This can be measured by assessing the highest point on the cornea that the inferior edge of the lens edge reaches on eye opening and then determining the lens movement to regain its position of rest. Ideally, postblink movement of lens should not be more than 1–2 mm along the vertical meridian and it should have a smooth movement across the corneal surface on the vertical direction. An alignment fit ensures smooth movement whereas in case of flatter fit, the movement is likely to be about the corneal apex. In highly toric cornea, the lens will have more erratic movement.

- Then examine the influence of upper and lower lid. A high positioned upper lid will not reach down on blinks to lift the lens to a central position. On the contrary, a tight lid tension could lift the lens too up. The lower margin is likely to support the lens and aid lens centration. Lower positioned lower lid will have minimal lens support (Box 5.1).

Static Fit

The assessment of the static fitting of RGP lens enables the practitioner to determine the relationship between the lens back surface and the anterior corneal surface. The assessment is done in the primary gaze position. The practitioner may manipulate the lens position to hold it at the center with the help of upper and lower lids. Now with the lens at the center, the fluorescein pattern is assessed and recorded to assess the following:
- Central fit
- Midperipheral fit
- Edge clearance or lift.

Central Fit

The areas of bearing or touch and clearance are assessed on slit lamp with cobalt blue filter. The dark area shows the areas of touch or flat fit, dark green area shows fluorescein pooling or steep fit, and light green

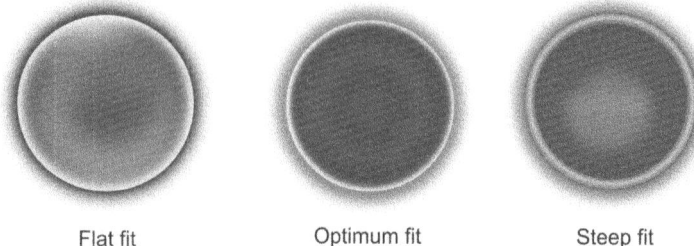

Flat fit   Optimum fit   Steep fit

Fig. 5.1: Rigid gas permeable (RGP) lens central fitting as shown by fluorescein pattern.

shows apical clearance or alignment. A well fit spherical RGP lens will show apical alignment of base curve over the pupil and bearing evenly distributed in the intermediate zone. A steep lens will show deep central pooling and a flat fit will touch the cornea as near circular black zone will be evident with no fluorescein. This is how the degree of fluorescein pooling may be graded as steep, slightly steep, and very steep and the degree of contact between the lens and the cornea can be graded as flat, slightly flat, and very flat.

Ideal fit will be seen as minimal apical clearance indicated by light green at the center, when observed in slit lamp as shown in Figure 5.1 (optimal fit). The central picture of Figure 5.1 shows ideal central fit with least pooling shown by dark color.

Midperipheral Fit

The midperiphery of an RGP lens is a very ill-defined zone. It is not exactly the midpoint between the center of the lens and its edge, as that point is well within the optical zone of the back surface in most of the cases. Midperipheral fit is an important part of an RGP lens fitting as RGP lens rests on the periphery.

A steeper lens fit will show dark area of fluorescein or area of contact at the midperiphery with central pooling or clearance at the center. A flat lens will show fluorescein spread around the midperiphery or lack of contact. When there is central pooling, a band of contact is observed adjacent to the zone of pooling as a dark area. The bearing area may be seen as a 360° band. When the central zone exhibits apical touch, i.e. flat fitting, the midperipheral fit should exhibit clearance from the cornea which is evident by the presence of fluorescein.

Ideal fit will be seen as minimal area of touch or bearing indicated by dark area in the midperiphery.

Edge Clearance or Lift

The second component of the peripheral fitting assessment involves the depth or clearance between the lens back surface and the cornea, i.e. edge clearance or edge lift. The amount of edge lift in the contact lens greatly influences lens positioning and is very important to facilitate tear exchange. As a general rule, the more edge lift a lens has, the more it will interact with the upper lid and too little edge lift will tend to have poor lid attachment and will ride low. Therefore, finding the right amount of edge lift can make the difference between fitting success and fitting disaster.

A greater edge lift increases the volume of fluid available for tear exchange and therefore, will exhibit dark green fluorescein pooling on a wide peripheral pattern, whereas a thin peripheral pooling indicates that the lens has too little edge lift. Too little edge lift will result in low-riding lens fitting and too much edge lift will result in high-riding lens fitting.

Ideal edge lift will be seen as light green band of 0.5–0.75 mm wide, when observed in slit lamp. The central picture of Figure 5.2 shows ideal edge lift as shown by bright peripheral ring (Box 5.2).

OVERREFRACTION

Once the lens fitting is optimally finalized, it is important to assess accurately the required back vertex power (BVP) with the trial lens in place. Prior to performing the overrefraction, the practitioner should

Box 5.2: TRAITS OF IDEAL STATIC FITTING OF RIGID GAS PERMEABLE (RGP) LENS.

- Minimal apical clearance indicated by light green at the center
- Minimal area of touch or bearing indicated by dark area in the midperiphery
- Light green band of 0.5–0.75 mm wide edge lift

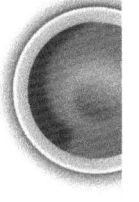 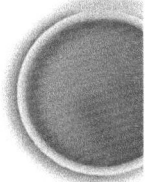 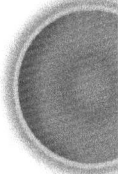

    High edge lift   Optimum edge lift   Low edge lift

Fig. 5.2: Edge lift in different fitting type.

take care to check the quality of the wetting of the front surface of the lens. If the lens wetting is poor, the end point of the overrefraction will be uncertain due to the irregular refractive surface.

If the trial lens wets poorly, it should be removed and rewetted by wetting solution, and then put back on the cornea.

Usually, overrefraction is done with spherical lens only. If the vision is unacceptable, a full spherocylindrical overrefraction is required if an unacceptable level of vision is obtained with spherical lens alone. The overrefraction result will dictate the BVP to be ordered. If significant cylinder is found, consideration of the need for toric RGP lenses is required. The ocular refraction at the corneal plane can be calculated from the spectacle prescription and the back vertex distance. The optical effect of the tear film should be considered. For example, on an eye of K reading 7.70 mm sphere, an RGP lens of 7.70 mm back optic zone radius (BOZR) is tried which appears loose due to poor lid support. Therefore, another RGP lens of 7.60 mm BOZR is tried that achieves a good fit. The positive power tear pool beneath this lens must be taken into account while calculating lens power to order and judging whether this is the power expected from ocular refraction.

A rough guide is that an RGP lens of BOZR fitted 0.10 mm steeper than flattest K reading will lead to a +0.50 D power tear pool. Therefore, an extra -0.50 D must be incorporated in the ordered lens power to neutralize this effect.

LENS ORDERING

Care must be taken while writing the RGP lens order for the patient. If the practitioner has a full understanding of the trial lens design, the written order is placed with all design features. Other characteristics of the lens such as the BVP, center thickness, material type, and tinting should be determined by the practitioner.

If the tears are relatively greasy or have mucous debris, good wettability and deposit resistance of the lens material is most important. The practitioner should avoid choosing lens materials that tend to attract lipids that would render the lens surface hydrophobic. Oxygen transmissibility is another criterion for choosing the lens material.

RIGID GAS PERMEABLE LENS PARAMETERS CHANGE AND LENS FITTING

In order to achieve a desired satisfactory RGP lens fitting, sometimes modifications as to the lens parameters may be necessary. An

understanding of the relationship between lens parameters is therefore, essential for the clinician to determine the clinical implication of any of the following parameter changes.
- Lens diameter
- Lens thickness
- Back optic zone radius
- Back optic zone diameter

Lens Total Diameter

Assuming other parameters remain the same, the change in lens total diameter may result in a flow-on-effect on the overall fitting. The change in total lens diameter affects the following aspects of the lens fittings:
- Lens centration
- Corneal coverage
- Lens movement/tightness
- Tear exchange
- Lens-lid interaction.

A reduction in lens total diameter affects both dynamic and static fitting of the lens as under:

Dynamic Fitting

- Loosen the lens fit
- Increases the lens movement
- Decentration is more likely.

Static Fitting

Reduces edge width and clearance, therefore, the fluorescein pattern depicts flat midperipheral fitting.

Larger diameter may be chosen to provide a larger optical zone for larger pupil diameter and also for lens stability. For every 0.50 mm increase in BOZD, there must be 0.05 mm increase in BOZR to maintain the same fluorescein fitting pattern.

Lens Thickness

Lens thickness is an important factor for lens stability on the cornea, if the BVP is more than 4.00 D. Thicker plus lenses are heavy and their center of gravity is on the front of corneal apex. Therefore, the lens will have a tendency to position low. Thinner lens edge also results in poor lens-lid interaction and favor low lens position. In such cases, a steep lens fitting provides the solution. Either smaller BOZR or larger BOZD will help.

In minus lens power, the center of gravity is posterior to the corneal apex and relatively thicker edges allow lids to grasp the lens and lift them to central position. This might lead to poor pupil coverage and uncomfortable lens fitting. Thin edges may minimize this problem.

Base Curve

A steeper lens fit produces a positive tear lens between the lens and the cornea, whereas a flatter lens produces concave tear lens between the lens and cornea. In order to compensate for the changes in the base curve, corresponding change has to be made in the BVP of the lens.

The thumb rule is a flattening by 0.05 mm produces -0.25 D effect which means lens power has to be changed by -0.25 D. Steepening by 0.05 mm produces +0.25 D effect which means lens power has to be changed by +0.25 D.

Example:
- RGP trial lens is fitted with BOZR 7.60 mm and BVP of -3.00 D. It is decided to change the BOZR to 7.70 mm; the new BVP would be calculated as under:
  Flattening by 0.05 mm produces -0.25 D effect. In this case, we are flattening by 0.10 mm.
  Therefore, the new lens BVP would be:
  $$-3.00 \text{ D} + 0.50 \text{ D} = -2.50 \text{ D}.$$
- RGP trial lens BOZR 8.00 mm and BVP of +8.00 Dsph, accurately corrects refractive error. The lens shows an apical touch fluorescein pattern on patient's eyes, so you decide to order a lens with same TD but with steeper BOZR 7.90 mm, new BVP will be calculated as under:
  Steepening by 0.05 mm produces +0.25 D effect. In this case, we are steepening by 0.10 mm. Therefore, new BVP will be:
  $$+8.00 \text{ D} - 0.50 \text{ D} = +7.50 \text{ Dsph}.$$

A change in BOZR without changing BOZD alters the central tear lens thickness as disclosed by fluorescein. The rule of thumb is for each 0.05 mm increase in BOZR, the BOZD must be increased by 0.50 mm to maintain the same sagittal relationship and central tear lens thickness.

In case of corneal astigmatism more than 1.50 D in which spherical lens is fitted, the BOZR should be decreased by 0.05 mm for each 0.50 D so that the corneal cylinder exceeds 1.50 D.

Back Optic Zone Diameter

When alterations to BOZD are made, the lens-to-cornea relationship and tear lens thickness changes. Increasing the BOZD causes an increase in the sagittal depth and therefore, greater central clearance. RGP lens with a larger BOZD will show a bright central pool of fluorescein, effectively making the lens fit tighter. Reducing the BOZD causes a decrease in the sagittal depth and therefore, greater central touch. RGP lens with a small BOZD will show a light central touch fluorescein pattern, effectively making the lens fit loose. Increasing the BOZD improves the lens centration and reducing the BOZD increases the lens decentration.

RGP LENS CARE AND MAINTENANCE

RGP lens material differs from the soft lens material in the sense that they are nonabsorbent in nature. They have hydrophobic surface properties. They are more rigid and durable than soft contact lens. Hydrophobic lens surface increases lens deposits. But the deposits cannot penetrate the lens matrix. They remain on the lens surface. Siloxane materials are more prone to proteins, whereas fluorine is more prone to lipids. This implies that RGP contact lenses are easier to care for than soft lenses, but they require different approach. Daily cleaners, storing solution, and disinfection are important. Alcohol base daily cleaners are more suitable for fluorosiloxane, which tends to acquire lipid deposits. Surfactants and protein removers are common cleaners used to remove deposits. Deposits can also be removed by repolishing the lens surface. Cleaning pads may also be used for the purpose. Care must be taken as aggressive cleaning may also damage the lens surface or change the lens power. Rinsing may be done with tap water, but it must be done with extensive caution. However, before lens insertion, rinsing should be done with soaking or storage solution. Only chemical system of disinfection is advisable as heat system will warpage the lens. Wet storage always increases the initial comfort. Dry storage or using a lens case with flat bottom may lead to lens warpage. Multipurpose solution serves the purpose of wetting, soaking, and disinfection. Hydrogen peroxide system is rarely applied for RGP care because of its poor wettability properties.

INSTRUCTIONS FOR RGP LENS INSERTION

- Put the wet and clean right lens on the tip of the index finger or middle finger of your dominant hand.
- Balance the lens on the tip of your forefinger.
- Now pull down the lower lid with the middle or ring finger of the same hand. Use your other hand to hold the upper lid together with lashes; open the eye firmly.
- Look directly at the lens or into a mirror and place the lens directly on cornea.
- Release your lower lid first and then slowly release your upper lid and then blink.
- Rotate the eye and the lens settles in its place or gently manipulate the lens by using the eyelids to center.
- Repeat the procedure for your other eye.

INSTRUCTIONS FOR RIGID GAS PERMEABLE LENS REMOVAL

- Look straight ahead and open your eyes as wide as possible.
- Put the fingertip on the outer corner of the eyelids so that pressure is applied to both upper and lower lid margins.
- Pull the finger toward the ear and slightly upward and open the eye as wide as possible.
- Bend your face down and keep your cupped hand under your eye.
- Blink strongly and hold the lens in your other hand.
- If the lens does not come out with the first blink, relax, reposition your finger, and repeat.

Spherical RGP Lens Fitting

MULTIPLE CHOICE QUESTIONS

Q. 1. The HVID of a patient is 11.80 mm; suggest the appropriate total lens diameter of the initial RGP trial contact lens for the patient.
  a. 9.80 mm
  b. 11.80 mm
  c. 13.80 mm
  d. 10.80 mm

Q. 2. Which of the following statement is relevant to consider while selecting lens diameter for RGP contact lens to a patient?
  a. Larger palpebral aperture is likely to need larger lens diameter.
  b. Larger lens diameter is indicated if lids are loose.
  c. Flatter corneas may need larger lens diameter.
  d. All of the above

Q. 3. Which of the following is not the trait of the ideal static fitting of RGP lenses?
  a. Minimal apical clearance indicated by light green at the center
  b. Minimal area of touch or bearing indicated by dark area in the midperiphery
  c. Light green band of 0.50–0.75 mm wide edge lift
  d. Heavy contact zone in the midperiphery of the cornea

Q. 4. Which of the following is the trait of ideal dynamic fitting of RGP lenses?
  a. Well centered and well stable lens
  b. Consistent lens movement with the change in position of eye gaze
  c. Smooth movement of lens with blink
  d. All of the above

ANSWERS

1. a   2. d   3. d   4. d

Q. 5. During the trial of RGP lens fitting, suppose you decide to reduce the total diameter of the lens only without correspondingly altering the BOZR, what could be the possible effect?
a. The altered diameter lens is likely to show increased lens movement.
b. The altered diameter lens is likely to show more lens decentration.
c. The altered diameter lens is likely to loosen the lens fit.
d. The altered diameter lens is likely to tighten the lens fit.

Q. 6. In RGP lens fitting, flatter corneas need .... lens diameter.
a. Same					b. Smaller
c. Larger				d. Steep

Q. 7. While fitting RGP lens, the omission of cylindrical component will be taken care of by the:
a. Cylindrical lens			b. Spherical lens
c. Tear lens				d. Toric lens

Q. 8. While fitting RGP lens, ideal edge lift will be:
a. 1.00 mm				b. 0.50–0.75 mm
c. 2.00 mm				d. 1.00–2.00 mm

ANSWERS

| 5. c | 6. c | 7. c | 8. b |

CHAPTER 6

Therapeutic Contact Lens Fitting

INTRODUCTION

Ophthalmologists have been using the contact lenses for years as therapeutic agent for the treatment of corneal diseases as drug delivery vehicle. With the introduction of extended wear soft lens, the use of therapeutic lenses has developed into a major modality of treatment for corneal disorders to promote wound healing, sealing of corneal perforation, and mechanical protection to cornea.

INDICATIONS

The applications of therapeutic contact lenses are indicated in cases where the need is felt to:
- Relieve the pain by covering exposed corneal nerve endings.
- Deliver the drug.
- Protect the cornea against abrasive effect of lids and promote the healing.
- Seal corneal perforation.
- Provide structural support to cornea.
- As an alternative to tarsorrhaphy.

However, care must be taken to rule out fitting therapeutic lenses in following cases:
- In cases where the cornea is already hypoxic, such as when there is anterior segment ischemia due to severe chemical burn.
- In cases where the eye is very dry and instillation of wetting solution is not enough to keep both the contact lens and the cornea hydrated.
- In cases where the cornea is very sensitive, as in some cases of corneal erosion, the patient will not be able to tolerate the contact lens.

OCULAR DISORDERS THAT CAN BE TREATED WITH BANDAGE CONTACT LENSES

The following common ocular disorders have been very frequently treated with therapeutic contact lenses:

Bullous Keratopathy

The treatment of choice for painful bullous keratopathy is to use an extended wear soft contact lens. The relief of pain is immediate and most patients will not allow their lenses to be removed unless a promise is given to reinsert the lens.

Exposure Keratitis

When the exposure is due to lagophthalmos or protrusion of eyeball, the use of soft contact lens as a bandage lens is contraindicated because of poor blinking. Tarsorrhaphy is the most effective way of treatment except in the following cases:
- In one-eyed patient, where tarsorrhaphy is not a suitable option.
- In case of bilateral keratitis where one cornea is already severely scarred.
- Where there is severe lid retraction.
- Where the patient refuses to undergo tarsorrhaphy.

The patient should be instructed how to clean and wear the lens when it is accidently dislodged. During sleep, lens should not be worn and a sticky tape can be used to keep the eyes shut. Use low water content daily wear, if possible, as they cause less dehydration. If rigid lens is well-tolerated, one can use a rigid gas permeable contact lens.

Corneal Ulcer

In some corneal ulcers where the healing is not observed in spite of adequate drug treatment, bandage lens may be tried. The lens acts as scaffolding for epithelial cells to heal over. High water content soft contact lens is the lens of choice.

Corneal Erosion

Most cases of corneal erosion respond to conservative treatment with pad and antibiotic eye drops. In some cases, extended wear soft contact lens can be fitted for a trial period. However, if the contact lenses are not tolerated, they should be removed immediately.

Corneal Perforations

In cases where the corneal perforations cannot be sutured surgically, the use of therapeutic lenses can be successfully done with extended wear soft contact lenses.

Corneal Injuries

Corneal burns, which do not heal with conservative treatment, can be treated with contact lenses. When pain is severe, a bandage lens is indicated.

Trichiasis

When conventional treatment fails, one can try using an extended wear soft contact lens. However, where dryness is an associated problem, frequent instillation of wetting solution may be required.

Postoperative

Following ptosis operation, an exposure keratitis may develop. This can be treated with an extended wear soft contact lens. Following pterygium surgery, when an extensive superficial keratectomy has been done, patients have severe pain for the 1st day or 2. In these cases, the use of a bandage lens can relieve pain. An extended wear soft contact lens can also be used following keratoplasty. Post-photorefractive keratectomy (post-PRK) patients are also benefited with soft extended wear bandage lens.

OTHER THERAPEUTIC INDICATIONS

In the following cases also, use of therapeutic lenses are indicated:

Orthoptics

Contact lenses are also used as occluders in the occlusion therapy for amblyopia and in the relief of diplopia.

Corneal Irregularities

Where there are corneal surface irregularities causing irregular astigmatism, due to injury or disease, they can be best corrected with rigid contact lenses.

Unsightly Eyes

Tinted contact lenses can be used to cover up unsightly corneal scars or opacities, due to various causes. Soft lenses can be color printed, hand printed, or can be colored like iris. They can be designed with a clear and opaque pupil.

Photophobia

Tinted contact lenses can also be used in aniridia and albinism to reduce photophobia. Pinhole contact lens can be used in polycoria.

Orthokeratology

This is the practice of the reduction of refractive error by altering the shape of the cornea with contact lenses. The shape of the cornea can be flattened by increasing flatter contact lenses.

FITTING CRITERIA

The fitting of bandage lenses is very simple. Because they are large and soft, the standard bandage lenses can mold to the shape of most cornea. Keratometry is not necessary and in most cases not possible. The lenses are also highly gas permeable and can be used for extended wear of time. The following care must be taken while fitting therapeutic lenses:

- In case of dryness, avoid using high water content lens.
- In case keratometry is not possible, follow the other eye.
- In case of corneal graft or limbal inflammation, lens diameter should be 14.50–16.00 mm.
- Cover the patient with antibiotics as the risk of infection is high, especially in diabetes and dry eyes.
- For long-term cases, provide the patient with a spare lens in case of loss.
- Avoid the use of contact lens where the eye is hypoxic or dry or hypersensitive.
- If the eye cannot tolerate extended wear, try a daily wear lens.

THERAPEUTIC CONTACT LENS CARE AND MAINTENANCE

Care and maintenance of therapeutic lenses require some extra precautions. Always use clean and lint-free hands while handling lenses and in cases of perforated cornea insist on sterile procedure. See the patient the next day, and regularly thereafter. Instruct the patient to consult you, if there are any unusual eye symptoms. Also inform relevant consultants, if thin lenses are fitted as they may be overlooked.

Teach the patient or his companion how to remove the contact lens, if required. There is no need to teach how to insert the lens, as he should have his eye examined by you before reinsertion. A new lens is always better than a lens that has to be cleaned and reinserted.

Multiple Choice Questions

Q. 1. In which of the following case the fitting of therapeutic contact lenses is not recommended?
   a. Relieve the pain by covering exposed corneal nerve endings
   b. Protect cornea against the abrasive effect of lids and promote healing
   c. As an alternative to tarsorrhaphy
   d. In case where cornea is very sensitive, as in some cases of corneal erosion

Q. 2. Which of the following statements is true with regards to SiHy therapeutic contact lenses?
   a. Uncomfortable on painful eyes
   b. Low modulus
   c. Decreased risk of SEALS
   d. Increased water content

Q. 3. Which of the following is not a main function of therapeutic contact lenses?
   a. Relieving pain
   b. Correction of refractive error
   c. Mechanical protection and support
   d. Maintenance of corneal epithelial hydration

Answers

1. d   2. a   3. b

CHAPTER 7

Presbyopia and Contact Lens Fitting

INTRODUCTION

Presbyopia correction with contact lenses is highly challenging and rewarding for the optometrist and is a compromise for the lens wearer. The two additional factors, which are very critical for successful fitting of presbyopic contact lens, are as following:
1. Careful selection of lens design
2. Managing patient's expectations

The main types of contact lens for presbyopic correction are:
- Monovision correction
- Enhanced monovision
- Alternating or translating lens design
- Nontranslating or simultaneous vision lens design.

MONOVISION CORRECTION

Monovision correction is the technique in which one eye is corrected for distance vision and the other eye for near vision. Usually, dominant eye is corrected for distance vision and nondominant eye is corrected for near vision. Monovision practice is an ideal option for occasional user of contact lenses. It requires less chair time to fit and the success rate is reasonably good, if the patient is adequately educated. While educating the monovision wearer, educate the patient to insert the near lens first and remove the near lens last. They are simpler to fit and less expensive than the bifocal lenses. The other side of monovision correction is the reduction of stereopsis and contrast sensitivity, which creates a question mark on patient satisfaction. The need for blur suppression is also an issue.

ENHANCED MONOVISION

One eye can be fitted with single vision lenses and the other with bifocal lenses or both eyes may be fitted with two different designs. A variety of fitting philosophy may be thought of:

- The most common practice philosophy is fitting the dominant eye with single vision distance correction and the nondominant eye with bifocal contact lenses.
- Single vision near lens can be fitted in dominant eye to improve near visual performance and a distance bias bifocal contact lens can be fitted in the nondominant eye.

The practitioner dynamic approach is the key to decide the suitable philosophy for a patient.

ALTERNATING OR TRANSLATING VISION LENS DESIGN

Alternating or translating lens design is similar to the spectacle bifocal lenses. The superior portion is designed for distance vision and the inferior portion for near vision. The patient must look through two separate portions to see either near or distant objects. Both near and far cannot be seen clearly at the same time. They are executive type segment, have visible demarcation line, and are gaze dependent. Straight gaze will allow him to see through the distance power zone and down gaze will provide him to see through the near power zone. Head and lid positions are critical for successful fitting of such lenses. Loose lids, lower lid below the limbus, and lower lid too far above the limbus are contraindicated for translating bifocal contact lenses. However, adequate translation and comfort on eye have always been an issue with this type of lenses.

NONTRANSLATING OR SIMULTANEOUS VISION LENS DESIGN

In case of nontranslating or simultaneous vision lens design, rays of light from distance, near, and all intermediate distances enters the eyes simultaneously. Vision is corrected in all directions of gazes. The retinal image so formed shows the whole range of objects present in the field of view. The patient has to select or concentrate on one or other. Currently, this is the most popular presbyopic option for contact lenses.

Broadly, there are three types of simultaneous vision lens design:
1. Concentric bifocal lenses
2. Diffractive lenses
3. Aspheric multifocal lenses.

Concentric Bifocal Lenses

Concentric bifocal lenses are simultaneous vision lens with two or more distinct regions of power. The distance and near areas are sharply defined and both the distance and the near vision portions of the contact lenses covers the pupil. It implies that the visual system needs to select the clear image at the required distance. Image clarity is relatively independent of pupil size. The drawback of this type of lens is that it is only a bifocal lens and hence intermediate vision is compromised. Ghosting or double vision is also an occasional problem.

Diffractive Lenses

Diffractive lenses are simultaneous vision multifocal lens developed in multiple circumferential Fresnel type design. It is really difficult to understand how it works as one must be familiar with the mathematics of light waves. The lens design is not dependent upon pupil size. Distance and near images are seen at the same time. Poor contrast is a big issue and hence not good for night driving. They might be good for people with moderate near addition.

Aspheric Multifocal Lenses

Aspheric multifocal lenses are simultaneous vision lens with gradual change in power from near to distance, i.e. the power gradually changes from the center to the edge of the optic zone much like progressive ophthalmic lenses. The distance and near areas are not sharply defined. The transition zone provides the correction for intermediate distance. At all times, the pupil is covered simultaneously by both the distance and the near vision portions of the contact lenses. The visual system, therefore, does the job of selecting the clear image at the required distance. The lens performance is pupil size dependent. The advantages of this type of lenses are no image jump, no ghosting of images, and vision is clearer at all distances.

In case of aspheric multifocal contact lenses, lens power is distributed concentrically. The overall lens power may be distributed with maximum near add in the center and all other power at the periphery or distance power at the center and maximum near add in the periphery.

Based on this, the aspheric multifocal lenses may be divided into two categories:

1. CD Aspheric (center of lens corrects distance vision)
2. CN Aspheric (center of lens corrects near vision).

INDICATIONS FOR PRESBYOPIC CONTACT LENS FITTING

The patient must fulfill the usual criteria for successful contact lens wear and in addition, the ideal patient for presbyopic contact lenses is one who can accept compromise in their distance and near vision and who is not very particular about vision clarity. Care must be taken to avoid emmetrope for distance and patients with cylinder power more than −0.75 D or −1.00 D, patient with high visual demands, patients who need good sustained close vision for near work, and who are poor at handling the lenses. Long-term users of contact lenses who do not wish to start wearing spectacles even for reading are motivated to go for presbyopic contact lens correction. Good motivation is the key to success.

FITTING METHODS FOR SOFT CONTACT LENSES FOR PRESBYOPIC CORRECTION

A mature and responsible patient would be more benefitted by presbyopic contact lens correction than an immature one. A comprehensive prefitting evaluation for fitting presbyopic contact lens must include the following:
- Spectacle lens prescription with near addition.
- Convert it to minus cylinder form.
- Vertexed in spherical equivalent prescription.
- Establishing the baseline binocular visual acuity at distance and near.
- Establishing the dominant eye at distance. Dominant eye is the eye that leads in fixation. Our visual system can suppress blurred foveal image better in the nondominant eye.
- Fit early presbyope with low addition in both eyes (up to +1.50 Dsph), whereas a mature presbyope often requires a high add for near vision (+2.50 and above).
- The challenge is fitting in between patients. For them, low addition is not enough for reading and high addition proves too much for them. Two separate additions may be thought to keep the patient binocularly happy. Low addition in dominant eye and high addition in nondominant eye is done (+1.75 Dsph to +2.25 Dsph).

- Also check lower lid laxity. Taut lower lid is essential and the position of lower lid should not be lower than the inferior limbus in order to support the lens.
- Pupil size evaluation is very important factor when fitting simultaneous vision multifocals as it is important information while selecting a presbyopic contact lens design. In general, pupil size reduces with age and there is less dilation of the pupil in presbyopic population in any given lighting condition. Working distance and patient's work place environment also affect the pupil size. Patient with small pupil will utilize and appreciate the add power better when using center near design multifocal lens. The change from near to distance power will also occur rapidly over the lens surface, allowing smaller pupil to utilize the full range of lens optics.
- Make sure that the pupil constricts in bright light and dilate in low light condition. If pupil does not constrict or dilate, it is quite likely that simultaneous vision multifocals may not be successful. For a CN lens design, the pupil needs to constrict to eliminate the distance portion of the lens from entering the pupil. Conversely, the pupil must be able to enlarge to allow the distance optics of the lens to enter the pupil as needed. If pupil dilation and constriction is not normal, the patient may not be a suitable candidate for multifocal lenses.
- Each type or design needs a specific approach for successful fitting, so it is always wise to follow manufacturer guideline for fitting.

INITIAL LENS FITTING EVALUATION

A trial lens fitting method is always good to manage the patient and establish the realistic expectations.
- Allow the lens to settle on the eye.
- Lens should center well and provide adequate movement.
- Assess vision assessment in normal illumination.
- Do not use refractor head or phoropter as shading effect of the instrument may dilate the pupil artificially.
- Use full aperture flipper or twirls to assess the over refraction.
- Binocular over refraction is preferable to monocular assessment.
- Use high- and low-contrast visual acuity chart to elicit useful idea with respect to possible success.
- For translating bifocal, the lens must move to ensure that approximately three-quarter of the pupil area is covered by the

correct section of the lens for both distance and near and the lens must move upward on down gaze to bring the near portion in front of the pupil area.
- Base curve selection has to be done as per manufacturer's guideline.

Multiple Choice Questions

Q. 1. Which the following patient is not expected to be the successful wearer of multifocal contact lenses?
   a. A patient who is highly motivated to use multifocal contact lenses
   b. A patient who is well counseled by the practitioner
   c. A patient who needs fine visual acuity for his daily routine work
   d. A patient who understands the importance of preset reasonable expectations from the multifocal contact lenses.

Q. 2. Which of the following patient is expected to be successful wearer of multifocal contact lenses?
   a. A patient with large cornea
   b. A patient with brisk pupil reaction
   c. A patient with flat corneas and laxity of lids
   d. High astigmatic patients

Q. 3: While looking at near object, what change happen in pupil?
   a. Pupil constricts
   b. Pupil dilates
   c. No change in pupil size
   d. Unrest

Q. 4. Use of which mirror is recommended while multifocal lens insertion?
   a. Concave   b. Convex
   c. Plain   d. Any

Answers

| 1. c | 2. b | 3. a | 4. a |

Chapter 8

Sports and Contact Lenses

INTRODUCTION

Contact lenses are one of the most important modes of vision correction in sports. While fitting contact lenses to athletes, it is to be remembered that contact lenses are not fitted to athletes but the athletes are fitted to contact lenses. The following considerations are important before fitting contact lenses to athletes and players:
- Sports and the position of athlete in the sports.
- Risk of trauma which may be very common in dynamic sports, e.g. soccer or hockey.
- Environment, for example, indoor environment usually is characterized by no air flow and low humidity.
- Relative risk of nonionizing radiations.
- Comfort issues which may be worst in non-dynamic sports when the eyes are static.

All these conditions must be considered in relation to the athlete's own physiology. In sports like swimming or sailing, the choice of correction may be combination of contact lenses and spectacle on top. In general, fitting contact lenses to athletes yield advantages has been shown in Figure 8.1.

PERIPHERAL AWARENESS

Nearly all sports demand good peripheral awareness. Possessing a relatively large field of vision is obviously asset in terms of sports

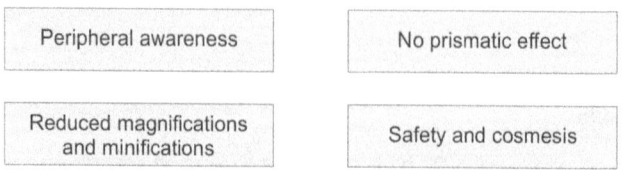

Fig. 8.1: Advantages of fitting contact lenses for athletes.

performance. There are two simple reasons. Nature and evolution have made us more sensitive to movements in the periphery area of field of vision. Typically, lots of conflicting movements are often present in our peripheral field of vision. It implies, therefore, in addition to seeing the peripheral area of field of vision, an awareness of the objects in the periphery is equally important. Since contact lenses move with eyes, they provide an excellent macular field of vision. On the contrary, glasses are paired with the frame where lens edge and the frame rim also limit the field of vision. In basketball and football, both offensive and defensive players must have awareness of where the ball is, where his teammates are, and where the opponents is at all time, suggesting that the larger range of field is a factor that greatly contributes to good sporting performance in these events.

NO PRISMATIC EFFECT

Observing through an eccentric zone of the lens creates a prismatic effect. A prismatic effect leads to deviation similar to heterophoria that the individual tries to compensate with his own binocular fusion. It may cause:
- Strain, if the deviation is moderate.
- Asthenopia or diplopia, if the deviation is greater. The result is observed as increase in fixation disparity or unstable fixation disparity which ultimately affects stereopsis adversely.

Since contact lens does not significantly decentralize with respect to the individual's visual axis, no undesirable prismatic effects occur. This is particularly important in case of anisometropia.

REDUCED MAGNIFICATIONS AND MINIFICATIONS

A minus spectacle lens makes objects in the field of view appear smaller; whereas, a plus prescription makes objects look larger in the field of view. These changes are further aggravated when the refractive error is significantly higher. This is due to the vertex distance. Sometimes, it may create difficulties for an individual to move about in his environment without considering a short period of adaptation. With contact lenses, however, the objects are not so much magnified or minified as they lie on pupillary plane. So, this is an important criterion to select a vision correction mode for an athlete. However, an athlete who is habituated to use spectacle may find it difficult to adjust to contact lenses when fine judgment of depth is required. As it can be seen in table tennis where timing of a top spin smash relies critically on the distance of the bat from the ball and half of a millimeter can have drastic effect on the timing.

SAFETY AND COSMESIS

Cosmesis is all about appearance and look. How an individual looks to him and others is important; this is natural and cannot be ignored. There is no right and wrong when it comes to cosmetics. Some people feel that they look good in spectacles, while others take spectacles as the stealer of their personality. If an athlete does not wear a correction modality just because he feels that he does not look good, it would defeat the whole purpose of dispensing. This seems true also as playing sport is a social activity as much as an expression of competitive needs. The mode of correction which is cosmetically not appealing will detract the pleasure of the game. Another perception that has been seen to dominate the people's mind is that a product that looks good also performs better. It is coincidence that sports frames have part of their appeal routed in their fashion appeal. Contact lenses have the intrinsic advantage of not affecting the natural appearance of the athlete. When soft lenses are used for swimming, they also give a degree of protection from chemicals in the water. As long as lenses are disposed off after swimming, chemicals absorbed by the lenses do not remain in contact with cornea any longer. Hence, it could be argued that this is an advantage of wearing clean daily disposable contact lenses for swimming.

The factors that influence fitting of contact lenses for athletes are given in Flowchart 8.1.

Type of Contact Lenses

Broadly there are two types of contact lenses:
- Rigid gas permeable
- Soft contact lenses

Flowchart 8.1: Factors influencing fitting of contact lenses for athletes.

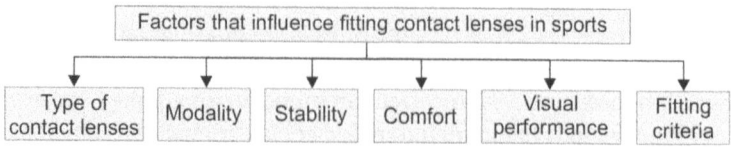

Rigid gas permeable lenses provide better visual acuity but the level of comfort is less as compared to soft contact lenses. There is an adaptation period of time which is quite significant and the wearer may feel the effect of glare and flare in dim light conditions. Soft contact lens improves peripheral vision and is more comfortable. Most wearer adapt to soft contact lenses very quickly. Soft contact lenses are the lenses of choice in sports.

Modality

The modality of contact lenses depends upon the duration of the sports and sporting environment. For example, in water sports like swimming or sailing, the first choice of modality is daily disposable lenses. Risk of acanthamoeba infection and chemical keratitis is unavoidable in swimming pool. The soft contact lenses absorb the contents of the water and if it is used for long, it could adversely affect, making daily disposable the lens of choice.

Stability

The need for stability affects the lens choice and fitting criteria. Soft contact lenses in fresh water (hypotonic) stick to cornea due to passage of water into the cornea and it floats away in salt water (hypertonic). This can be used to advantage in sports like canoeing, sailing, and water polo—as long as the lens sticks to right place. There are situations where contact lens may not be the correction of choice.

Comfort

Contact lens discomfort is a condition characterized by episodic or persistent adverse ocular sensations related to lens wear, either with or without visual disturbance, resulting from reduced compatibility between the contact lens and the ocular environment which may include eyes stinging, burning, itching, eye pain, abnormal feeling of something in the eye, and excessive watering of the eyes. Low humidity and no air flow in indoor environment may reduce wearing comfort. Static eye may also lead to reduction in lens wearing comfort.

Visual Performance

Contact lenses can affect contrast sensitivity, but this is far outweighed by the correction that can be achieved with them especially when the refractive error is small. Contact lenses are the ideal way of dealing with small refractive errors. Small cylinders can also lead to constant searching for clarity and spasm and can often be conveniently corrected by spherical contact lenses. Contact lenses are best for monocular refractive error correction. Strong dominant athletes find significant improvement in anticipation, i.e. to judge depth. However, care should be taken while fitting contact lenses as transient instability of vision post blink is critical in sports where static visual acuity is critical. Lose fitting lenses causes more decrement.

Fitting Criteria

Stability of contact lenses on the cornea is very important for accurate and undistorted vision. So, large diameter and steep fitting is advised for the duration of the game. Athlete may be informed that separate pair of contact lens needs to be used during sports which are not needed otherwise.

Contact lenses can be lost in many competitive contact sports especially some water sports where contact lenses can be contraindicated. Sport is not always clean and hands that get muddy or faces that get muddy make contact lens wear even more problematic. It is, therefore, important to consider the environment in which the athlete plays. Cold environments are often associated with low humidity, which in turn tends to induce lens dehydration. It suggests that low water content lenses will provide maximum resistance to lens dehydration. At high altitude, temperature falls and partial pressure of oxygen in the atmosphere decreases which suggests that High Dk/t lenses are essential for good ocular health. Rigid gas permeable lenses are prone to trap debris beneath the lenses and are clearly contraindicated in dirty and dusty environment. Aquatic environment is not suitable for contact lenses. Contact lenses are likely to increase the rate of infection. In fresh water chlorinated pool, there is a risk of Acanthamoeba infection. High water content lenses are contraindicated in marine due to salt environment.

Multiple Choice Questions

Q. 1. Which of the following contact lens has been suggested for swimming?
   a. RGP lenses
   b. Daily disposable soft contact lenses
   c. Monthly disposable soft contact lenses
   d. None of the above

Q. 2. Which of the following is not the reason for contact lens related discomfort?
   a. Low humidity
   b. No air flow in indoor environment
   c. Static eye
   d. Low altitude

Q. 3. Which of the following is the most important criterion for fitting contact lenses to athletes and players?
   a. Stability of contact lens on cornea
   b. Modality of contact lens
   c. Type of lens material
   d. Design of contact lens

Answers

| 1. b | 2. d | 3. a |

Chapter 9

Contact Lens Care and Maintenance

INTRODUCTION

The healthiest way to use contact lenses is to wear for 1 day, then remove and throw away prior to sleeping because there is no need to clean or store the lenses. Unfortunately, the most commonly prescribed lenses are ones that are used for some days and then disposed of on a regular recommended schedule. These lenses are taken out every night before sleep, cleaned properly, disinfected, and stored before they are worn again using appropriate lens care solution. Since contact lenses are in intimate contact with the eyes and are bathed in tears, they are prone to deposition with substances derived from the tear fluid, resulting in reductions in comfort, vision, and increased inflammatory responses. Microbial contamination is also possible during handling and storage.

Contact lens practitioner must prescribe appropriate lens care solutions together with the contact lenses and the prescription of solution has to be based on lens type and individual patient profile. The objective is to keep the lens clean, hydrated, and prevent microbial contamination so that the wearer can have consistent vision, enjoy wearing comfort, maintain the ocular health, and remain into the habit of wearing lenses. This is very important especially in case of reusable lens category.

Before prescribing a lens care solution, the practitioner must remember the fact that the main issues with soft hydrogel lenses are disinfection and protein removal. Hydrogel lenses may below water and non-ionic materials which may exhibit lower protein deposition. Hydrogel lenses may also be high water content nonionic, which may have potential for greater protein attraction because of higher water content. However, they have the advantage of nonionic polymer matrix that prevents additional interaction between protein and the lens. Low water ionic lenses have negatively charged surface that have a greater potential for positively charged tear proteins and lipids, whereas high water content ionic lenses attract more tear proteins.

Silicone hydrogel lens materials represent a whole new class of materials and behave entirely different from conventional hydrogel lenses. Most silicone hydrogel lenses are low water content, which means protein deposition is not a main issue. The main issue with silicone hydrogel lenses are enhancing surface wettability of the lenses and removing lipid deposition. Wetting agent has to be stronger in solution prescribed for silicone hydrogel lenses so that they hold water molecule for longer duration of time.

The care and maintenance of rigid gas permeable (RGP) lenses is slightly different. While the soft contact lens disinfecting solutions primarily have a single role, RGP disinfecting solutions are used for disinfection and enhancement of lens wettability.

The practitioner needs to prescribe appropriate solution and can recommend alternative products if a patient experiences difficulty while using lenses. This would be possible only when he has a fair knowledge of properties of the solutions which are determined by the compositions of the solution. Table 9.1 shows some of the components of a solution:

While recommending care and maintenance regimen, the practitioner should spend some chair time educating the patient regarding following:
- An approximate of 10 mL solution is consumed every day in cleaning and storing contact lenses. This implies 60 mL solution is for 6 days' use and 300 mL solution is meant to be used for 30 days. For tours and travels, 120 mL solution is good.
- All solutions when opened should always be kept tightly closed. Open or improperly closed cap may allow CO_2 entry in the solution which may make the solution acidic. Patient may report burning and stinging for some time. Also, there may be the possibility of microbial contamination.
- A contact lens bottle when opened should be finished within 90 days of its opening. This is in line with the instructions given on most medicines packaging. It means that they are to be followed for better results and sometimes for preventing harmful effects. It is quite likely that disinfecting properties of the solution may decrease over a period of time and in such the case it may increase the risk of infection by not performing as desired. Hence, it is better to discard the solution after 90 days of opening.
- Similarly, the practitioner should also talk about the expiry date of the solution and must explain that the properties and effectiveness

TABLE 9.1: Components of a solution.

Factors	Implications
Chelating agent	All solutions contain the chelating agent EDTA, which is antimicrobial preservative and an agent that may prevent lens deposits. This in turns enhances disinfecting ability of contact lenses.
Buffer	Buffers keep the pH near that of natural tears and enhance cleaning effectiveness. Average pH of tears is 7.00–7.40, which is in the state of neutral. If it is more than neutral state, the solution becomes alkaline and if less the solution becomes acidic. Initial discomfort as burning or stinging is noticed, if pH of the solution is beyond the range.
Surfactants	Surfactants remove deposits and debris from the lens surface. They also decrease the wetting angle of the lens material by changing surface energy and thus act as wetting agent. Every surfactant is wetting agent, but every wetting agent is not surfactant.
Preservatives	Preservatives are added to prevent microbial growth in the solution after opening. They also act as disinfecting agents for contact lenses to eliminate microorganisms from contact lenses. They are most common cause of toxic reaction or solution sensitivity. The disinfecting agent should be harsh on bacteria and genteel on eyes.
Demulcent agents	Demulcent agents are added to solutions to enhance water retention and surface lubrication of contact lenses. They also increase surface wetting of the contact lenses, and thus in turn increases contact lens wearing comfort.
Viscosity	High viscous solution keeps the lens hydrated for longer duration of time. They are good for dry eyes or dysfunctional tear syndrome. However, high viscous may leave runoff residue on the eyelashes or lids as solution dries out which may cause pathogen growth.

(EDTA: Ethylenediamine Tetraacetic acid)

of the solution may change with time and for this reason they should be used before the expiry date.
- Fresh solution should always be instilled every day to store the lenses and patients should be warned against any "topping up" of solution.
- Avoid transferring solution from one bottle to another. It is not likely that you can safely transfer the solution to another bottle without contamination.

- Avoid touching the tip of the solution bottle with fingers.
- The practitioner must demonstrate the exact procedure of using lens care solution. And when the patient comes for routine aftercare visits, he must ask him to demonstrate the way he uses lens care solution for regular lens care. A regular communication in all after care visit is the key to good patient compliance.
- "Do not change solution brand until I prescribe". This is an important statement that the practitioner must make while dispensing contact lenses.

Multiple Choice Questions

Q. 1. Which of the following is likely to cause lens-induced ocular discomfort?
 a. Solution-induced toxicity
 b. A steep fitted lens
 c. Use of daily disposable lens
 d. A well edge designed lens

Q. 2. What is the importance of buffer in contact lens solution?
 a. Buffer improves the wettability of the lenses
 b. Buffers keep the pH of the solution near that of natural tears
 c. Buffer enhances the disinfecting ability of the solution
 d. Buffer enhances the viscosity of the solution

Q. 3. Which of the following statement is true for the viscosity agent in solution?
 a. Higher viscosity may lead to accumulation of residues on eyelashes and lids
 b. High viscous solutions are good for dry eye cases
 c. High viscous solution may cause more pathogen growth
 d. All of the above

Q. 4. Using cleaners on the lens may render the surface more:
 a. Hydrophilic
 b. Hydrophobic
 c. Photophobic
 d. Photophilic

Answers

1. a   2. b   3. d   4. a

Appendices

APPENDIX 1: Vertex distance calculation chart for contact lens fitting [for back vertex distance (BVD) of 12 mm].

For minus read left-right		For plus read right-left	
−	+	−	+
5.00	4.75	10.25	9.12
5.12	4.87	10.50	9.25
5.37	5.00	10.75	9.37
5.50	5.12	11.00	9.62
5.62	5.25	11.25	9.75
5.75	5.37	11.50	10.00
5.87	5.50	11.75	10.25
6.00	5.62	12.00	10.37
6.12	5.75	12.50	10.75
6.37	5.87	12.75	11.00
6.50	6.00	13.00	11.25
6.62	6.12	13.50	11.50
6.75	6.25	13.75	11.75
6.87	6.37	14.00	12.00
7.00	6.50	14.25	12.25
7.12	6.62	14.75	12.50
7.37	6.75	15.00	12.75
7.50	6.87	15.50	13.00
7.62	7.00	15.75	13.25
7.75	7.12	16.25	13.50
7.87	7.25	16.75	13.75
8.00	7.37	17.00	14.00
8.12	7.50	17.25	14.25
8.25	7.62	17.62	14.37
8.50	7.75	18.00	14.50

Contd...

Contact Lens Fitting Guide

Contd...

For minus read left-right		For plus read right-left	
8.75	8.00	18.12	14.75
9.00	8.25	18.50	15.00
9.25	8.37	18.75	15.25
9.50	8.62	19.00	15.50
9.75	8.75	19.50	15.75
10.00	9.00	20.00	16.00

APPENDIX 2: Keratometry conversion table. (n = 1.3375, Cx surface)

6.50	51.92	7.80	43.27
6.55	51.53	7.85	42.99
6.60	51.14	7.90	42.72
6.65	50.75	7.95	42.45
6.70	50.37	8.00	42.19
6.75	50.00	8.05	41.93
6.80	49.63	8.10	41.67
6.85	49.27	8.15	41.41
6.90	48.91	8.20	41.16
6.95	48.56	8.25	40.91
7.00	48.21	8.30	40.66
7.05	47.87	8.35	40.42
7.10	47.54	8.40	40.18
7.15	47.20	8.45	39.94
7.20	46.88	8.50	39.71
7.25	46.55	8.55	39.47
7.30	46.23	8.60	39.24
7.35	45.92	8.65	39.02
7.40	45.61	8.70	38.79
7.45	45.30	8.75	38.57
7.50	45.00	8.80	38.35
7.55	44.70	8.85	38.14
7.60	44.41	8.90	37.92
7.65	44.12	8.95	37.71
7.70	43.83	9.00	37.50
7.75	43.55		

(Keratometers actually measure radius of curvature of cornea.)

Bibliography

1. Contact Lenses: Fundamentals and Clinical Use
By Harold A. Stein, MD, FRCS(C)
Melvin I. Freeman, MD, FACS
Raymond M. Stein, MD, FRCS(C)
Lynn D. Manad, BA, CLS

2. Soft Contact Lenses: Clinical and Applied Technology
By Montague Ruben, FRCS, DOMS

3. Contact Lenses: Procedures and Techniques
By Gerald E. Lowther, OD, PhD

4. Contact Lenses: Medical Aspects
By M Ruben, FRCS, DOMS
C Y Khoo, FRCSE, FRACS, DO, AM

5. The Contact Lens Manual: A Practical Guide to Fitting
By Andrew Gasson, FCOptom, DCLP, FAAO
Judith Morris, MSc, FCOptom, FAAO, FIACLE

6. The Complete Contact Lens Fitting Guide and Directory
By Joseph W Soper, FCLSA
Peter R Kasti, MD, PhD

7. Contact Lenses: A Guide to Successful Wear and Care
By Prof. Hikaru Hamano
Prof. Montague Ruben, FRCS, LRCP, DOMS

8. A Textbook on Contact Lens Practice
By Devendra Kumar, FBCO, DCLP (UK)

9. Questions and Answers on Contact Lens Practice
By Jack Hartstein, MD

10. Contact Lens in Ophthalmic Practice
By Mark J Mannis, MD, FACS
Karla Zadnik, OD, PhD
Cleusa Coral- Ghanem, MD, PhD
Newton Kara-Jose, MD, PhD

11. Contact Lenses: Advances in Design, Fitting, Application
Edited
By Joseph W Soper

12. Contact Lens Practice: Visual, Therapeutic and Prosthetic
By Montague Ruben, FRCS(Eng), DOMS(Eng)

13. IACLE Resource Materials

14. Eye Dominance in Sport: A Comparative Study
By Geraint Griffiths, BSc Mech Eng, MSc Optom, MC Optom

15. The Incidence of Ametropia in Elite Sport
By Geraint Griffiths, B Sc Mech Eng, M Sc Optom, MCOptom.

Index

Page numbers followed by *b* refer to box, *f* refer to figure, and *t* refer to table

A

Accelerated stability design 55, 56*f*
Allergy 17
Aspheric multifocal lenses 79, 80
Astigmatism 48
   against-the-rule 49
   classification of 49, 49*t*
   corneal 49
   internal 49
   irregular 49
   lenticular 49
   oblique 49
   regular 49
   residual 49
   total 49
   with-the-rule 49

B

Back central optical radius 6
Back optic zone
   diameter 27, 67, 69
   radius 6, 50, 66, 67
Back up lens available 2
Back vertex power 33, 48
Bandage contact lenses 74
Base curve 5, 6, 61, 68
   radius 6
   selection 42
Bifocal lenses, concentric 79, 80
Bi-weekly disposable lenses 2
Blending 5, 8
Blink rate 17, 25, 28
Bullous keratopathy 74
Burns, corneal 75

C

Central posterior curve 6
Color cosmetic contact lenses 4
Conjunctiva 16, 21
   examination of 21
   function 21
   normal 21
   observe 22
   rule out 22
Contact lens 1, 3, 9, 11, 13, 73, 75, 84, 88, 90
   back optic zone diameter of 27
   care 90
   case cleaning 38, 39
   classifications 1
   design variables 4, 5*f*
   fitting 16, 78, 95
      contraindications for 29
   for athletes, factors influencing
      fitting of 86
   induced acute red eye 29
   maintenance 90
   material 13
      general properties of 10
   power 9
   surface 12*f*
   types of 86
Cornea 16, 20
   curvature of 48, 96
   examination of 20
   function 20
   normal 20
   observe 20
   rule out 20
Corneal coverage 34, 67
   assessment of 34

Corneal curvature 25
  measurement 17
Corneal diameter 25, 26
  measurement 17
Corneal erosion 74
Corneal hypoxia 10
Corneal injuries 75
Corneal irregularities 75
Corneal perforations 75
Corneal sensitivity 17, 25, 28
  test 29f
Corneal ulcer 74
Crystalline lens 48

D

Daily disposable lenses 1
Diffractive lenses 79, 80
Dispense lens 42
Double slab off stabilization design 55, 55f
Dry eye
  soft contact lens fitting in 44
  symptoms 23
Dry spot 24

E

Edetate disodium 40
Elasticity, modulus of 13
Enhanced monovision 78
Ethylenediamine tetraacetic acid 92
Eye 9
Eyelashes 16, 19
  examination 19
  function 19
  normal 19
  observe 19
  rule out 19
Eyelids 16, 18
  examination 18
  function 18
  normal 18
  observe 18
  rule out 18

F

Fitting contact lenses for athletes,
  advantages of 84f

Fitting disposable soft contact lenses 44
Fitting silicone hydrogel lenses 41
Fitting soft contact lenses 32
  fitting methods 32
  indications 32
Fitting soft Toric lenses 48
Flattening lens 9
Fluorescein 32
  staining 20, 21

G

Good soft contact lens fit, traits of 37b

H

Heat-based disinfection procedure 39
Horizontal visible iris diameter 26, 33, 60
  measurement 26f
Hydrogen peroxide 43
  based system 40
Hydroxyethyl methacrylate 3
Hydroxypropyl methylcellulose 39

I

Immunosuppressive drugs 30
Infection 23
Initial base curve 33
  selection 60
Initial lens
  fitting evaluation 82
  power selection 60
Iris color 17, 25, 29

K

K reading 60
Keratitis, exposure 74
Keratometer 25, 96
Keratometry 76
  conversion table 96
Keratoplasty 75

L

Lens
  and prescribed solution package 42
  back vertex power of 48
  centration 35, 67

Index

delivery 37
design, careful selection of 78
diameter 67
final cylinder axis of 53
fitting 66
intolerance 23
lid interaction 67
mislocation 51
movement 35, 36f, 67
ordering 66
power selection 61
rotation 50
   compensating for 53
   measuring 52
thickness 67
tightness 35, 67
total diameter 67
   selection 60
Lid
   angles 56
   eversion 16, 22
      examination 22
      normal 22
      observe 22
      rule out 22
   lens interaction 36
   margins 16, 19
      examination of 19
      function 19
      normal 19
      observe 19
      rule out 20
   tension 56
   tonicity 16, 25, 28, 61
Lipid layer thickness 25
   assessment 25
Lower lid, position of 56

M

Midperipheral fit 63, 64
Monovision correction 78
Monthly disposable lenses 2
Movement test 42

N

Narrow beam examination 20, 21
Noninvasive tear break up time 23

O

Ocular disorders 74
Optical zone 5, 7
Orthokeratology 76
Orthoptics 75
Overrefraction 57, 65
Oxygen
   permeability 10
   transmission through lens 11f

P

Palpebral aperture 17, 25, 27
   size 27f, 61
Photophobia 76
Poloxamine 39
Poor lens fit 23
Post-photorefractive keratectomy 75
Precontact lens fitting eye examination 16
Presbyopia 78
Presbyopic contact lens fitting,
      indications for 81
Presbyopic correction 81
Preservative-free lens care products 44
Prism ballast 54, 54f
Pupil diameter 17, 25, 27, 27f
Push up test 36f

R

Refraction 17, 25, 29
Rigid gas permeable lens 3, 22, 59, 66
   care and maintenance 69
   central fitting 64f
   ideal dynamic fitting of 63b
   ideal static fitting of 65b
   insertion, instructions for 70
   removal, instructions for 70
Rose Bengal test 23

S

Schirmer test 23
Silicone hydrogel lens 3, 41, 42, 91
   care system 43
Simpler lens care 2
Simultaneous vision lens design 78, 79
Skin, modified folds of 18
Slit lamp observation 21t

Sodium fluorescein 24
Soft contact lens 3, 32
   care system 38
   fitting methods for 81
   parameters, altering 37
Soft hydrogel lenses 3
Soft lens
   insertion, instructions for 44
   removal, instructions for 45
Soft Toric lenses 48
   use of 48
Solution, components of $92t$
Spherical corneas 32
Spherical rigid gas permeable lens 48
   fitting 59
Spherocylinder over refraction 50
Sports and contact lenses 84
Superpermeable contact lenses 41

T

Taco test 44
Tear
   break-up time 23, 24
   exchange 67
   film 17, 23
      examination of 23
      function 23
      normal 23
      quality 23
   lens 9, $10f$
   prism height 23, 24
   thinning time 23, 25
   volume 23
Therapeutic contact lens
   care and maintenance 76

fitting 73
use of 75
Tissue damage 23
Toric lens 50
   fitting, vertex calculations in $51f$
   trial 57
Toric orientation laser marks $52f$
Toric soft contact lens 49
Toric stabilization design, selecting 54
Total lens diameter 33
   changing 37
   factors affecting $61t$
Trial lens
   back vertex power of 33
   fitting method 32
   selection 34, 62
Trichiasis 75

V

Vertex distance calculation chart 95
Vertical palpebral aperture, size of 56
Vertical visible iris diameter 26
   measurement $26f$
Vision
   better 2
   correction 29
   lens design
      alternating 78, 79
      translating 78, 79
   reduced 23
   stability 37
Visual performance 87

W

Wide beam examination 20, 21

EU GSPR Authorised Reprsentative
Logos Europe, 9 rue Nicolas Poussin
1700, La Rochelle, France
Phone: +33 (0) 6 67 93 73 78
E-mail: contact@logoseurope.eu

www.ingramcontent.com/pod-product-compliance
Ingram Content Group UK Ltd.
Pitfield, Milton Keynes, MK11 3LW, UK
UKHW021303180426
11947UKWH00015B/995